Dedication

This book is dedicated to my wife, who has stood by my side (even when I didn't deserve it) and has continued to love me deeply and unconditionally, and to my daughter Natalie, who just makes every day delightful. Both make me a better Christian, father, husband, friend, and doctor.

Thank you, and I love you.

D0288374

About the Author

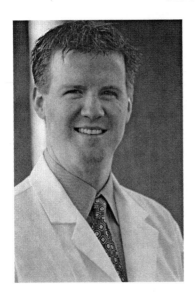

Brent Stewart, M.D., M.B.A. was born and raised in Arkansas. He attended Arkansas State University where he received an undergraduate degree in zoology. He then obtained his medical doctorate degree from the University of Arkansas and served a 4 year anesthesiology training residency at the University of South Florida. Later, he earned a masters degree in business administration from the University of Florida. Dr. Stewart became board certified as an anesthesiologist in 2007.

www.NeedSurgeryNowWhat.com

Foreword

"I don't want to know anything; I don't want to feel anything." I have heard this so many times, and I understand it completely. While I do this every day, surgery is a completely foreign experience to you. You're anxious, and you didn't sleep well last night. You woke up at 5:00 a.m., and you skipped breakfast. On top of that, you're wearing a tacky gown in an uncomfortable bed, waiting to turn your body and mind over to a guy you just met. It doesn't seem like the best way to start your day.

I always appreciate when patients share these concerns, and it often happens. It is a constant reminder of how frightening the surgical process can be, and how much trust you place in me. You may be one of several patients I'll see today, which is just another day in my regular week. But this may be your first surgery. And even if it's not, you're still nervous. Beyond that, you're important. You're somebody's <u>one</u> mother. Somebody's <u>one</u> father. Somebody's big sister. Somebody's little brother. Somebody's *sweetie*. It's a privilege taking care of you, and I promise I'll care for you like you were in my family. I know surgery and anesthesia can be scary, but part of that fear comes from lack of information. So, I have written this text hoping that you will learn some new information that will put you more at ease.

The surgical process can be much less frightening and much more pleasant if you are prepared from a knowledge and mental attitude standpoint. That is the purpose of this book. This text contains important information that should make your surgery a more positive experience.

Approach to the Book

If you're preparing for surgery, you probably don't want to read a long book, particularly if much of the material is unrelated to what you're having done. So, I encourage you to read about the Types of Anesthesia, Drugs, Lines (because you may get one), and What to Expect. Then, just read the information specific to your surgery. I want you to be <u>informed</u> but *not* <u>overwhelmed</u>.

If you're interested, I have added more information generally about being a doctor and specifically about the medical professionals who administer anesthesia. If you wish, read about all of the different types of surgeries. Read a little. Read a lot. I just want you to get comfortable with what to expect. Make it *your* book.

Always ask a qualified physician before taking medications or relying upon any provision of this book on a specific basis. This book is intended to provide information that you can use to better understand and participate in your surgical care decisions. It is not intended as a substitute for your physicians or their team members. It does not constitute an informed consent. Please do not take any action, medication, or make any decision based solely upon this book. Please confer with your physicians before taking any action or making any decisions with respect to your health care or the health care of anyone else.

What is anesthesia?

Simply put, anesthesia is the lack of sensation. But anesthesia is a spectrum, and it can mean anything from numbing the skin to complete unresponsiveness in surgery. It is a balance of "sleepiness" against the degree of surgical stimulation. Ideally, the "depth" of anesthesia should counterbalance the stimulation of the procedure. That is, the more something hurts, the more anesthesia you need to cover it.

Rendering an anesthetic requires us to manipulate and manage your physiology. In fact, we maintain the physiology while the surgeon rearranges the anatomy! We use monitors and drugs to provide the right amount of anesthesia, while minimizing side effects. We find that perfect balance, the right amount of medication, under these circumstances, at this time, for this patient: you.

Top 10 Questions People Ask Before Their Surgery

1.   Will someone be with me during my entire surgery?

Good question. In fact, several patients have asked whether we just administer a shot and then leave the room. I suppose many people think that. After all, they're asleep, so how would they know otherwise?!

The answer is yes. Someone trained in anesthesia will constantly be with you. You will not be left alone in the operating room. As you will read later in the book, anesthesiologists work with two types of mid-level providers: anesthesiologist assistants (AA's) and nurse anesthetists (CRNA's). This is just like your surgeon who may have a physician assistant (PA) or a nurse practitioner (ARNP).

In some hospitals, there are only anesthesiologists. There, the anesthesiologist stays in the room the entire time. Elsewhere, anesthesiologists work as a team with these mid-level providers. In such a case, the anesthesiologist is 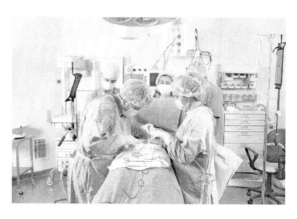 involved in putting the patient to sleep, and the AA or CRNA stays with the patient during the case. Understand that, like flying a plane, the *planning* of an anesthetic is the greatest challenge. Once the surgery is underway, a mid-level provider is capable of continuing the anesthetic. The anesthesiologist is always available for any questions or issues that may develop. Notice in the photo that everyone's attention is focused on the patient. That's the way it is and how it should be.

2.   Are you sure that I will wake up? How long will it take?

In short, yes. It is extremely uncommon for a patient to die in surgery. Our anesthetics are very safe, and we have a lot of training in how to use them. In fact, the incidence of death is about

1 in 200,000. Furthermore, if we think that a patient is high-risk, then we usually delay surgery until the patient's condition is improved by specialists. What that means is that, if we think you are at risk for death in the OR, then we won't take you there. Also, anesthetics don't typically create new problems. Healthy patients have very little about which to be worried.

Of course, we cannot predict the future, and bad things happen. An unanticipated difficult airway could present itself, or a patient could have malignant hyperthermia, a condition explained in the Special Considerations section. These are very rare. One of the best things you can do to protect yourself is to openly discuss your medical history and concerns with your anesthesiologist.

In most circumstances, patients wake up a few minutes after the surgery is completed. When anesthesiologists talk about waking up, we mean that the patient is following commands and breathing well. Since some of our medications normally cause amnesia for a time after surgery, patients may not be able to form memories immediately after the surgery. So, a patient may think that he didn't wake up until a couple of hours later, but, in fact, he did. Unless special circumstances occur, the wake-up from most anesthetics occurs shortly after the procedure is finished, even if there is no memory of being awake at that time.

3.   <u>Will I remember anything?</u>
The short answer is "no". The longer answer is "no or probably not". We understand you don't want to remember anything, and it's our intention to make it that way for you.

If you have a general anesthetic, then you won't remember anything after you go to sleep. That is, you won't wake up in the middle of your surgery. Understand that remembering the ride down the hallway, the entry into the operating room, and the monitors' being connected is perfectly fine. "Awareness" under anesthesia is an extremely rare occurrence, and it is discussed further in Special Considerations.

If you are to only have sedation, then remembering things like lights and voices in the OR is OK. The purpose of sedation is to simply "take the edge off". While most people still don't remember anything in this case, having vague recall of voices or other sounds does not indicate a problem. We will make it so that the experience is not bothersome.

4.   <u>Will I get overdosed?...or underdosed, for that matter?</u>

We have several monitors to evaluate your depth of anesthesia. We monitor your heart rate, blood pressure, and respiratory rate, among other things. Changes in any of these can tell us how to adjust the anesthesia. Our experience, combined with vigilant assessment of these parameters, assure that you will get the right amount of medication.

Think of an anesthetic as a bucket. All we have to do is fill the bucket. We can fill it with one drug or smaller amounts of multiple drugs. The combination that will work for you is best decided by you and your anesthesiologist. Considerations such as your age, current medications, body size, surgical position, medical problems, and your desired wake-up-time are things for the two of you to discuss.

5.   <u>Will I be nauseated?</u>

We are very aggressive about preventing nausea, so probably not. But, it depends on the type of anesthesia and surgery. If you have just some sedation, then nausea is extremely uncommon. If you need a general anesthetic, then nausea is *a bit* more likely. Also, if you have a problem with motion sickness, then nausea is more common. Certain procedures and certain anesthetics can make the risk higher. But we have several medications that can lower the risk. Please discuss your concerns with your anesthesiologist, and you can refer to the Special Considerations section for more information.

6.   <u>How much pain will I have?</u>

Most people should expect a little discomfort, and that's it. Some patients may have a nerve block (Regional Anesthesia) that provides complete pain relief after surgery. For the remainder of patients, we give enough pain medicine under anesthesia that the patient wakes up with just a little tenderness. We are very good at knowing the right amount of medicine to administer. Furthermore, pain medicine is also given in the recovery room as you wake up. We won't let you be in excruciating pain. If you have a history of issues with pain management, please let us know so that we can design an intelligent pain relief plan for you.

7.   <u>I've heard about a tube in my throat. What is it? Will I have a sore throat?</u>

You *might* have a sore throat. But first, let's clear up a couple of things. One: you may not have to have the tube. We don't use it if we're simply going to sedate you. Two: you're asleep when it is placed. Except for the fact that some people ask about it, most don't ever know it was there.

The purpose of the tube is to protect your airway and to provide breathing for you. Some anesthetics require a breathing tube. That's because the medications we need to give you for your surgery will cause your breathing to weaken, and so we must take over. Other times, the breathing tube is helpful because we need to get out of the surgeon's way. We want to maintain good breathing, but we can't interfere with the surgeon. As examples, consider surgeries on the mouth, nose, and brain.

Understand that there are two "pipes" in the neck. One is the windpipe (trachea), and the other is the food pipe (esophagus). The windpipe goes down into the lungs, and this is the pipe in which we put the breathing tube (like shown in the picture). It passes the vocal cords to get into the trachea, which is why some people will have a sore throat. The soreness usually goes away in about a day. Throat lozenges are usually enough to deal with any discomfort. So, *if* you have a general anesthetic and *if* you have a breathing tube between the vocal cords, then you *might* have a sore throat. (There is another type of "tube" that doesn't go between the vocal cords. Soreness with it is rare.)

8.   <u>Will I say something silly while I'm "under"?</u>

Boy, that would make for some good stories, right!? Sadly, no, you won't. Most *patients* want to be very sleepy, and most *surgeons* want the patients very sleepy! That's because a chatty patient might serve as a distraction to the surgeon. So, don't expect to be awake enough to be talkative.

Oftentimes, while you're waiting to go into the OR, you will get some sedation. It's not enough for the surgery, but it helps you to relax. Right *then*, you might be silly, but we are going to give you more medicine when the surgery is underway. If you can make it into the OR without giving out PIN numbers, signing blank checks, or telling family stories, then your secrets should be safe!

9.   What is the OR like?
        Basically, it's a large, bright room. And it tends to be rather chilly. There are bright lights, lots of equipment, and a narrow operating table. If you get a little sedation before surgery, as many people do, you won't remember going in there. But a picture is worth a thousand 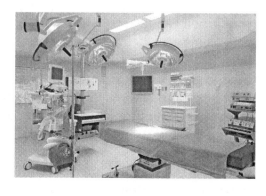 words...and so I'll spare you. Most look something like the photo.

10.   What are the long-term effects of anesthetics?
        First, long-term negative effects from simple sedation (MAC) are unlikely. Second, with regional anesthesia, permanent nerve injury is possible, but it is extremely rare. Since spinal and epidural injections require that the needle pass through strong back muscles, soreness can result. Third, general anesthetics *can* have neurologic effects in patients older than 60 years. We have learned that there *can* be some decline in cognitive function (ability to concentrate, for example) after general anesthetics. The effect is temporary, and it is often discovered only with sophisticated neurologic testing.
        While such potential side effects may be alarming, they should not dissuade patients from undergoing surgeries that are necessary. Obviously, no one has surgery just for fun. If you need to have multiple surgeries with general anesthesia, then the possibility of cognitive decline should not get in the way. Rather, a thorough discussion with your anesthesiologist will lead to an intelligent anesthetic design that will allow you to have your surgical issue addressed and to do it in a way that minimizes side effects.

What are the types of anesthesia?

There are several varieties of anesthesia. Let's start with the simple ones and work our way up the spectrum in complexity.

Local anesthesia

A local anesthetic actually has a double meaning. To some, it means that the anesthesia, or numbing medicine, is placed locally - under the skin, for example. This is done for a small area, and it refers to WHERE you put it. To others, a local anesthetic is a type of medication. It refers to WHAT you are putting. To an anesthesiologist, it is both. If a doctor were going to take out a splinter or place stitches, he would use a local anesthetic (the WHAT), and he would place it in or near the wound (the WHERE). With simple local anesthesia, there is no sedation. Only the skin is numbed. Local anesthetics are often used in minor office procedures, such as removing a mole or having a dental procedure. For information on allergies and local anesthetics (particularly for Novocaine), please read the Allergies section in Special Considerations.

Regional anesthesia

A regional anesthetic is the application of a local anesthetic (the WHAT) to a group of nerves to make a *region* (the WHERE) go numb. A regional anesthetic covers a larger area than a local anesthetic. Two of the most common regional anesthetics are spinals and epidurals, which are often used for Cesarean sections and laboring mothers, respectively. However, there are bundles of nerves all throughout the body. Commonly anesthetized bundles of nerves are found in the neck, armpit, groin, and back of the thigh. We call these regional anesthetics "nerve blocks".

The purpose of numbing a nerve or nerve bundle is pain relief. In addition to pain relief *after* surgery, a regional anesthetic can help *during* surgery, too. Consider... How much sleeping anesthesia would it take to amputate a hand? A lot! Now, how much sleeping anesthesia would it take to amputate a hand *if* the hand and arm were first made *completely* numb? None! Because there would be no feeling in the arm, the surgery could be performed with the patient wide awake or with sedation or all the way asleep, whichever the patient preferred. A numb body part means you need less brain anesthesia. Less brain anesthesia means fewer side effects and a faster wake-up. The combination of a regional anesthetic (like a spinal or certain nerve blocks) and sedation can be a very elegant approach.

A regional anesthetic requires the placement of a needle into a specified area. There are four main risks associated with that. The first risk is unintended bleeding. If you are on blood thinners (aspirin is OK), you are probably not a candidate. Blood thinners can obviously make bleeding worse. We typically avoid bleeding in a place where we can't see it and stop it. Second, there is also some risk of infection, though we always thoroughly clean the site. So, an infection at the needle site is unlikely. Third, there is a risk of injury to nearby structures. Human anatomy isn't always identical to the textbooks. Sometimes our needles will touch an unintended structure. The fourth risk is that we could injure the nerve we're trying to numb. Remember, the whole point is to get very close to a nerve in order to effectively numb it. Injury is rare. (Generally, the worse the risk, the less likely it is to occur.)

The above explanation is not intended to frighten the reader or discourage the acceptance of a regional anesthetic. On the contrary, nerve blocks are very commonly performed and are extremely useful. For completeness, the common risks are provided along with the usual benefits. Your anesthesiologist will explain these risks further and answer any questions you have.

Monitored Anesthesia Care (MAC)

Moving along in the anesthesia spectrum, we come to a middle ground. This middle ground has had a few names in the past, including "twilight", "sedation", or "conscious sedation". When patients say they want one of those, we know what they mean, but we call it a "MAC". If they really, really want a lot of sedation, we call it a "big MAC"!

MAC is the state of sedation under which you will still respond to stimulation. That's not necessarily as bad as it sounds. We have a variety of medicines to keep you comfortable. In smaller doses, all of them will allow you to respond. Responding does not mean remembering. That's an important point.

The wake-up from a MAC is typically quick. We do not use a breathing tube, and the risk of nausea is small. For the appropriate patient having certain types of procedures, a MAC is a very nice way to minimize anesthetic side effects and promote a rapid discharge from the hospital.

General anesthesia

This is the most well-known type of anesthesia, and is the "deepest" kind of anesthesia. During a general anesthetic, you typically have a breathing tube (after you go to sleep), and you do not respond to surgical stimulation. From your perspective, the anesthesia begins and ends in an instant. In adults, the anesthetic is initiated by an IV injection. Children go to sleep by breathing the anesthesia.

During the surgery, the anesthesia is adjusted based on the degree of surgical stimulation. For example, surgical stimulation is more intense during surgery than for the suturing at the end of surgery. During those stimulating times, we will do the right thing to make sure that your body remains asleep, comfortable, and stable. Rest assured, someone trained in anesthesia, who can make those appropriate adjustments, is always in the room.

At the end of surgery, we stop giving the medications that keep you asleep. That's how you wake up. That's why we talk about the drugs "wearing off". Once you can follow commands (squeezing my hand, for example), we pull out your breathing tube. No one really remembers this. You may have a sore throat, but this usually resolves within 24 hours. There can be some discomfort after surgery, but excruciating pain is quite rare. Nausea is possible, but medications are routinely given to minimize this risk. Of course, your anesthesiologist and recovery nurse will quickly address any problems or difficulties if they arise.

Drugs

We use drugs to induce and maintain anesthesia. It is the combination and amounts of drugs that allow us to design an anesthetic that makes sense for you. Below are some common examples.

Opiates (narcotics)

Common opiates are morphine and fentanyl (pronounced FENT-a-nil). There are several others. Oral opiates, which we do *not* use in the operating room, include oxycodone and codeine. Opiates are excellent pain relievers. They will cause you to relax, and they may even make your nose itch! Opiates do not harm any organ; they are extremely safe in this regard. These are very effective drugs, and the side effects are mild when used properly.

Opiates also reduce the amount of other drugs you need to be given. They do not cloud your mind, but they may make you sleepy. In large doses, these drugs will cause pronounced heart rate slowing, lowered blood pressure, and slowed breathing. Excessive doses will cause breathing to stop, which is why these drugs should be given with supervision. Additionally, they are famous for causing nausea. ALL OPIATES cause nausea. Some are worse than others. Morphine and codeine are notorious for this. Understand that this is not an allergy to these drugs. Given in the right amounts, opiates are almost always a great choice.

Sedatives

We commonly use Versed (Hoffmann-LaRoche), pronounced VER-sed. This is in the same family as Valium (Hoffmann-LaRoche), Xanax (Pfizer), and Ativan (Wyeth Pharmaceuticals), among others. We like Versed because it causes amnesia. Most patients are apprehensive about the anesthesia and surgery, and they appreciate a little relaxing medication. If we give them Versed, they can still be awake and calm, but their brains have a hard time forming memories. So, after surgery, they will actually tell us that we put them to sleep even before going into the OR. Not so! They just don't remember going in there!

For this class of medicines, there are some things to consider. First, since the amnestic effect can last beyond surgery, many patients still do not form memories until several hours after having the procedure completed. Second, patients who take these medications regularly and people who drink alcohol regularly may not have the amnestic effect from Versed and will probably require higher doses. Third, older patients, usually over the age of 65, may get confused after having received one of these medications. Several older patients have told me that they did not like the disorientation that they felt as a result. In these patients, I often opt to avoid this class of medications. However, there is nothing wrong with these medications, and, for many patients, they are excellent choices.

Propofol

This medicine was made famous by its intense media coverage in 2011. So, the medicine scares some people. Please don't be afraid of it.

It is pronounced PRO-po-fall. While opiates are considered pain medicines and Versed is a relaxant, propofol is a true anesthetic. Propofol, like opiates, is what I call a "clean medication". It takes effect quickly and wears off quickly with little residual effect. It does, however, require supervision by someone trained in its use. Propofol is commonly used for colonoscopies and other quick procedures done under MAC. Since it works so quickly, it is also used to induce a general anesthetic. Propofol is very commonly used in anesthetics.

Ketamine

Ketamine is the closest thing we have to a complete anesthetic. It induces anesthesia, and it provides intense pain relief. It also promotes good breathing and maintains the blood pressure. However, some people will say they had an out-of-body experience with ketamine. They were "dissociated" from themselves. They may report strange visions or dreams. This should make perfect sense when I tell you that ketamine is a derivative of PCP, or Angel Dust.

Since many anesthesia drugs will cause airway obstruction (bad snoring or even sleep apnea), ketamine is a wonderful drug for the patient who would have a problem with this. Additionally, ketamine opens up the lungs nicely, so it's also good for patients with COPD or asthma. In patients who are very sick, ketamine will maintain a good blood pressure. However, ketamine doesn't wear off quite as quickly as some of our other medicines, and some people do report those unusual visions as a side effect. So, it is less commonly used. Still, it has been my "go to" drug on several occasions, and certain patients do very, very well with it.

Gas

Here come the jokes about the anesthesiologist who sits around passing gas! It's true that most general anesthetics are administered with an anesthesia gas. Although it's not used anymore, an example of this gas is ether. We use gas to regulate the depth of anesthesia: the more stimulation involved in your surgery, the more anesthesia gas you will need. In addition to the agents like ether, we can also use nitrous oxide (laughing gas). Waking up from the general anesthetic happens when the patient breathes *out* enough of the gas he's been breathing *in*.

Muscle Relaxants (paralytics)

For *some* (*not all*) general anesthetics, we give muscle relaxants. The other term is "paralytic", but that sounds frightening. They are simply IV medicines that chemically relax the body's muscles.

In certain surgeries, they are necessary. The abdominal muscles, for example, are very strong. If those muscles aren't relaxed, then the surgeon can't close up the belly! Sometimes, this relaxation is necessary to keep the patient still during very delicate procedures such as brain surgery. These medications are given regularly and are nothing to fear. They're used to keep you safe.

News stories have reported on the rare cases of patients who were "paralyzed" with these drugs, but who did not receive enough of the anesthetics to stay asleep. This is called awareness. We are trained to avoid this, we have monitors to help detect it, and we regularly verify that our anesthetics are given in appropriate amounts. More information on awareness is provided at the end of the book, but know that it is exceedingly uncommon. Remember, in many surgeries, these medicines aren't even given at all!

Invasive "Lines"

The purpose of a "line" is to sit in either a vein or artery and perform some desired function. A "line" is a convenient word for a catheter. It's not the kind that goes in the bladder, but simply a tube that sits in a blood vessel. In fact, a standard IV could be called a "line". If we need to give certain fluids or monitor some element of physiology, we may put a big IV "line" (a.k.a. central line) in a vein. If it's important to monitor blood pressure or blood oxygen, we may place a "line" in an artery (a.k.a. arterial line). The type of surgery and your underlying medical conditions will determine what needs to be used. In the large majority of cases, sedation is provided before any lines are inserted. Therefore, most people aren't bothered by and may not even remember the line placement.

Central Line

A central line is simply an IV that sits in a large vein. Veins in the hand are bigger than those in the thumb, right? And veins in the arm are bigger than the ones in the hand. It makes sense that, as we go back toward the heart, veins get bigger. As we get closer to the heart, the veins are more "central" (as opposed to more peripheral). So, when we put an IV, or "line" in a close-to-the-heart, "central" location, we have a central line! Common places to put central lines are the neck (internal jugular vein), under the collarbone, or in the groin. In the photo, the central line is in the right internal jugular vein.

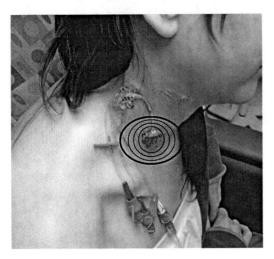

There are a variety of central lines. Depending on our needs, we will put in the appropriate line. The three-port (triple lumen) line, shown in the photo, is good for infusing multiple medications at the same time. The two-port (double lumen) allows us to administer fewer medications, but much more fluid because each of the two ports is bigger. The single-port (introducer) allows us to give lots of fluid and will let us "introduce" a fancy monitor called a P.A. catheter.

So, a central line has several benefits. It can monitor physiology from inside the body, facilitate the administration of multiple medications simultaneously, and allow blood draws for lab work (no more needle sticks). Also, it won't "fall out" like some peripheral IV's do. Placing one involves risks, like in everything else. Risks include bleeding (do you take blood thinners?) and infection (but we clean the area and work in a sterile environment). We can also damage nearby anatomy. Your anesthesiologist will explain further, but the risks are small.

Separately, you may have heard of a PICC ("pick") line. It is a Peripherally-Inserted Central Catheter, and it is placed in the underside of your arm. The catheter works its way through the peripheral veins into the central veins, hence the name. It is useful for long-term IV medications, and it won't "fall out" as peripheral IV's can. While it does not have all of the benefits of a central line, it also does not have many risks.

Arterial Line

An arterial line looks like an IV. It is typically placed on the underside of the forearm, just behind the thumb,

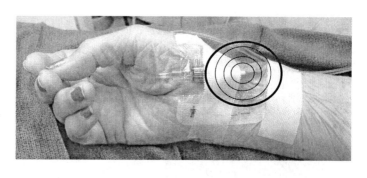

where you can feel your pulse. It sits in that artery, measuring your blood pressure with every heartbeat. It yields some very useful information. Additionally, we can draw blood from it that tells us how well your body is working with respect to oxygen and other factors. An arterial line is useful for procedures in which tight blood pressure control is important and for patients who are very sick.

What should you expect on your day of surgery?

Don't eat or drink anything after midnight. We know it's no fun, particularly if you have a late morning or, worse yet, an afternoon surgery. However, we need to avoid a condition called aspiration. Aspiration occurs when stomach contents, which are bathed in a very strong acid, get accidentally refluxed into the mouth and down into the lungs. The lung tissue is very delicate, and the hydrochloric acid in the stomach can do some serious damage. We have protective reflexes that keep the acid where it's supposed to be. But, when you get anesthesia, you lose those reflexes. There is a greater chance for the acid to get into the lungs. That's not good.

Unless otherwise instructed, please take your normal medications, except blood thinners and diabetes medicines. When I see you in the morning, I want you to be the same physiologic, chemical person that your primary care doctor has made you. If you fail to take your normal blood pressure medicines, you could have a pressure of 200/120, which is dangerous and could force a postponement of your procedure. How is that helpful to you or me?

We ask you to avoid blood thinners or diabetes medicines for specific reasons, as well. For diabetes medicines, it is logical that if you haven't eaten, you don't need anything to lower your blood sugar. Skipping breakfast will lower your sugar on its own! As far as blood thinners, they will make surgical bleeding worse. They also increase the risk of some regional anesthetics and central line placements. Understand that patients take blood thinners because they have heart stents, a prosthetic heart valve, an irregular heart beat, a history of stroke, or some other condition. Before you stop a blood thinner, make sure you have the approval of the doctor who originally prescribed it.

Next, expect a lot of paperwork. Expect people to ask you the same things multiple times. Expect to wait. Taking care of you is complicated. There are many things involved, most of which you will never see. Paperwork is a necessary evil. To ensure the proper procedure is done on the proper patient in the proper way, we will ask you many times. Please, please don't try to add a little spice to our lives by confusing us. I've seen a patient do that, and the staff was none too impressed. We have dedicated ourselves to taking

21

care of you, we and are taking your surgery very seriously. Even the simplest procedure still has checklists and safety requirements. All of that takes time. We want to get your surgery done and send you on to recovery as quickly as possible, but we won't compromise your health or safety to do so.

You must have an IV. There are exceedingly rare situations in which this can be avoided, but do not expect to be one of those exceptions. IV's come in different sizes, and a small IV is not always the best. Small IV's hurt (a little) less going in, but they tend to hurt more when you are receiving medication. Giving IV fluid is also slower through a small IV. When you get an IV, request some numbing medicine below the skin to make the IV placement nearly painless. It's a local anesthetic! Remember that from earlier?

You might be offered some pre-operative sedation, Versed. It is very common. This is in the same family as Valium. Kids can drink it, and adults get it through the IV. It causes amnesia and relaxes you. Please know that it may slow your wake-up a bit. In elderly patients the effect is more pronounced, occasionally causing confusion and excessive sleepiness.

The operating room is bright and usually a little chilly. Not to worry: you will get warm blankets. After the monitors are connected, you will breathe some oxygen through a mask. IV medications are given, and then you're asleep!

After surgery, you are taken to the recovery area, also called PACU. This unit is dedicated to the waking up of surgical patients. Here, the nurses are trained to recognize any problems related to surgery and anesthesia. You will receive more pain medicine, more anti-nausea medicine, or anything else you may require. If you received preoperative sedation, you may not remember being in this area, even though you were awake.

If you are to go home, then you can expect the nurse to go over instructions with you and your family. You may need to go by the pharmacy to get some medication. Don't worry about remembering anything. Your family is with you. This is a time for you to relax and recover.

If you are staying in the hospital, you will be transferred to your room when you are more awake. Your surgeon will write orders to take care of your medications, wound care, and diet.

Again, your only job is to relax and recover. Please let the nurses know if you need anything.

Within the first 24 hours, if you have a problem you suspect that is related to your anesthetic, please ask to speak with the anesthesiologist. Uncontrolled pain or nausea are examples. Outside of 24 hours, problems are not typically due to the anesthesia. Your anesthesiologist can also answer any questions regarding IV's, sore throat, or vital signs.

And now...

Anesthetics for Certain Procedures

Appendix

The appendix is near the junction of the small intestine and the large intestine (colon). We typically leave it alone unless it becomes inflamed, a condition called appendicitis. This oftentimes presents as pain in the right lower area of your belly, and you can see the small, worm-shaped appendix in the lower left side of the drawing. The image is drawn as if you were looking at someone else, which is why it is on the left side of the picture.

Usually, it is treated as an emergency. The most common surgical approach is laparoscopic (using cameras). Surgery to remove it is called an appendectomy (pronounced APP-en-DECK-to-me). Several small holes are made, and they usually close nicely. Most patients go home the next day. 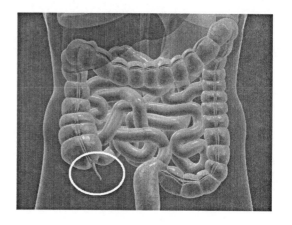 The alternative approach is to open the abdomen. Some patients will need this because they have had multiple abdominal surgeries or perhaps because the laparoscopic attempt is too difficult. The open approach is rare.

For the surgery, plan to have a general anesthetic. Other considerations during abdominal surgery are a function of your underlying medical problems. For example, a patient who has been vomiting for two days will likely have an electrolyte imbalance and dehydration, which will require an additional large IV. A very sick patient may need an arterial line to monitor changes in blood pressure. Your anesthesiologist will discuss this with you. There are several possibilities, and the ones just mentioned are common considerations.

Nausea is possible after abdominal surgery. If you have a history of motion sickness or nausea during a previous surgery, please let your anesthesiologist know. He can provide several medications to minimize this risk.

Arm and Forearm

Except for small surgeries on or just under the skin, the discomfort associated with procedures in this area can be significant. This is particularly the case when bones are involved. Still, complex surgeries that just involve tendons and muscles can be uncomfortable after surgery. For these cases, we often offer nerve blocks. Again, a nerve block is the application of a numbing medicine to a group of nerves to render a particular region of the body numb (and usually weak).

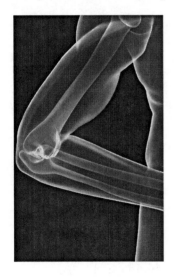

You are given sedation in combination with a nerve block, so you probably won't even remember it. Afterward, you can receive whatever kind of anesthesia you wish. Since you won't feel the surgery, you can have nothing, a little something, or a complete knock-out. Most patients don't have any interest in being awake (even if they don't remember it later) during surgery. The simplest thing for us to do, then, is to put you all the way to sleep with a mild general anesthetic. It's a very elegant way to have your procedure. The wake-up is quick, and there typically is no pain for 12-18 hours. The discomfort that comes later is much less intense and can be treated with pain pills.

Barring the use of blood thinners, infection in the area, or your refusal, a nerve block is a great way to have pain relief to the arm. If you don't want a block, which is fine, we will administer a general anesthetic, and you will receive IV pain medicine so that you wake up as comfortably as possible.

Back

Back surgery is often a last resort for patients who have suffered through pain injections, physical therapy, and daily narcotic use. Examples include laminectomies and fusions. Because of the history of narcotic use, you will require more pain medicine to be comfortable after surgery. Be very honest with your anesthesiologist about how much you are taking, as he will use that information to decide how much is the right amount for you.

These surgeries require a general anesthetic. They can last several hours and, depending upon the difficulty and duration of the procedure, there can be significant blood loss. Your anesthesiologist may place an arterial line to monitor your blood pressure, and he may plan to give you blood. If you have religious or other personal preferences regarding blood, please make that clear to the anesthesiologist, surgeon, nurses, and staff.

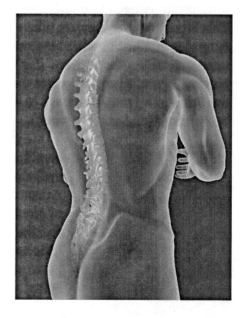

For patients having much smaller back surgeries like a kyphoplasty (KI-fo-PLAS-tee) or a vertebroplasty (ver-TEE-bro-PLAS-tee), the anesthesia can be MAC. These procedures involve using live X-ray to carefully place needles into a bone or a space. The skin is numbed, and with some IV sedation, the procedure is done relatively quickly.

Birth, Labor Epidural

A labor epidural is a type of regional anesthesia (discussed earlier in the text). The epidural is a source of angst for many mothers. Some women feel strongly that they should not have one. Perhaps they feel that the epidural will dull the labor experience for them. For whatever reason, they should not feel bad if they choose to pass on the offer. Similarly, women who would like to have one should not feel that they are somehow less of a person or are in some way harming the baby. They are not. This procedure is purely a matter of choice.

Most epidurals have no apparent complications. However, risks of an epidural include headache (usually starts 2-3 days after the epidural is placed), back pain (there are strong muscles in the back that can get inflamed), bleeding, infection, and nerve injury (very rare). Of the risks, the headache is the most common. Treatment includes lying down, lots of fluids, some caffeine, and pain medicines. Many times, the headache goes away in a couple of days. If it doesn't, your anesthesiologist can treat it if you return to the hospital.

An epidural is placed in the low back in a space called the "epidural space", hence the name.

To clear up any misunderstandings, <u>the spinal cord does not go all the way to the natal cleft ("butt crack")</u>. Try this. Put your hands on your hips. The tops of those bones on your sides are called the iliac (ILL-ee-ack) crests. They are at the level called L3,4. The spinal cord *ends* about 2 bony levels (~3 inches) higher than that. We place our epidural needle at L3,4 (top of your hips). Therefore, it is *impossible* to hit the spinal cord when placing an epidural or spinal at L3,4. That is the number one fear of patients, and now you know better!

Most anesthesiologists prefer to have you sitting for an epidural. An alternative is to lie on your side. Go with whatever the anesthesiologist is most comfortable doing. You will need to curl up like the letter "C",

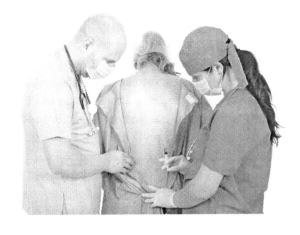

a mad cat at Halloween, or a shrimp. Pick your image, and mimic it. This helps open up the spaces in the back. I realize this is a difficult position when you're contracting and when you have a big baby belly! Your nurse will help you. Do not be afraid. The skin and tissue below are numbed first, and then you should just feel some pressure. The initial numbing stings a little bit. Once the epidural is in, you will get some medicine through it. The epidural space is not quite next to the nerves, so it takes a few minutes to get really numb. By the time the paperwork is done, you will probably be all smiles.

Birth, Cesarean section (C-section)

Please read the above section on Birth, Labor Epidural. Both a labor epidural and a spinal are types of regional anesthesia (discussed earlier in the text).

There are three types of anesthetics for C-sections (C/S): spinal, epidural, and general. Know also that there are two scenarios for C-sections: emergency and elective. Let's take each scenario in turn, discussing the different anesthesia approaches.

The **emergency** C/S occurs when a laboring mother or her fetus gets into trouble. If Mom already has an epidural, we can use it. Alternatively, the anesthesiologist can pull out the epidural catheter and quickly place a spinal anesthetic. It only takes a few moments, and the anesthesia is complete (no "hot spots"). Your anesthesiologist will suggest what he thinks is most appropriate for you.

Stated another way, if your epidural is working wonderfully, it's fine to continue using it for a Cesarean section. You get to skip another stick and have your baby. If the epidural isn't perfect (maybe you are still hurting a bit), then consider a spinal anesthetic. You typically want to avoid a general anesthetic. Heartburn, lung physiology changes, breast engorgement, and weight gain of pregnancy make a general anesthetic (all the way to sleep) less ideal in these situations, particularly for the mother who would like to hear her baby's first cry!

Next, the **elective** C/S is done for patients who have had previous C/S and for patients who do not need or do not want to have a trial of labor. Since it is elective, the morning proceeds the same as for other elective surgeries: no breakfast, lots of paperwork, etc. Almost universally, you will have a spinal anesthetic. A spinal is the ideal anesthetic for these cases, as it allows you to be awake for the baby, provides complete pain relief (you will feel pressure as the baby is taken out), and minimizes the general anesthesia risks mentioned above.

A spinal block is closer (than the epidural) to the nerves that are to be numbed. In fact, the medicine is placed into the fluid that surrounds the brain and spinal cord (it's called CSF). The drawing shows the needle tip in the CSF. <u>Remember that there is no spinal cord at this level, so direct injury to the spinal cord is impossible!</u> The numbing with a spinal occurs within seconds. Lowered blood pressure and nausea are also possible and normal. Treatment is straightforward. A headache can

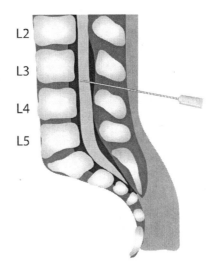

develop a couple of days later. It doesn't happen a lot, and it often improves with fluids, caffeine, and rest. Relax, wait for your husband to arrive in the room, and prepare for that first cry! ...the baby's, not yours!

Understand that because the spinal medicine lasts about three hours, expect to have numb, weak legs for a couple of hours in the recovery room. The nurses will be assessing your baby in the newborn nursery, so this will be a good time for you to sleep. When you wake back up, your legs should be awake. This may be one of your last uninterrupted nap times. Enjoy it, and good luck!

Bladder, cystoscopy (looking in with a camera)

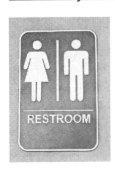

A cystoscopy is the use of a camera to look into the bladder by way of the urethra. It is as uncomfortable as it sounds, and so simple sedation oftentimes is not enough. Passing the camera into the bladder can be stimulating, and so a solid anesthetic is warranted. There are two options. The first consideration is the general anesthetic. This is frequently done. In this case, you are completely asleep during the procedure. There is a slight risk of nausea associated with a general anesthetic, but medications can significantly reduce that risk. The second option is a spinal anesthetic. The spinal anesthetic is nice because it allows you to be minimally sedated (or moderately, if you prefer) and very comfortable. After the spinal is placed, you do not feel any part of the surgery. However, the drug commonly used in spinals will last approximately 3 hours. You may find that a 2-hour wait in the recovery room, during which time you cannot move your legs or eat anything, to be both boring and distressing. Still, in some patients it is a good (and even preferred) option.

After the surgery (and after the spinal wears off), there isn't a lot of pain, but there may be a sensation of needing to urinate. This is particularly the case if a urinary catheter (we call it a Foley) has been left in place. Please note that a review of a spinal (regional) vs. a general anesthetic can be found earlier in this text.

Bladder, stimulator

A stimulator is used for patients who have difficulty controlling the bladder. It is placed in stages, first with a trial. In each of these procedures, it is important for your urologist to be able to communicate with you. So, the anesthesiologist balances a mild degree of sedation for your comfort against your surgeon's need to talk with you about how well the stimulator is working. Furthermore, you will be lying on your stomach, so we must be careful not to make your body too sleepy. Understandably, the thought of being "awake" in the operating room is daunting. But know that sedation is provided so that the patients actually do quite well, and the surgeons use a numbing medicine so that the procedure is not very painful. As in most things, the thought is much worse than the actual procedure.

Blood vessel (major vascular)

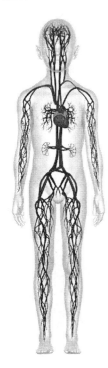

Common surgeries of this type include AAA (abdominal aortic aneurysm) repair and fem-pop (femoral-popliteal) bypass. These are large arteries, found either in the middle of the abdomen or in the groin. Patients who have problems with these large arteries tend to also have problems with other arteries, namely the arteries of the heart (coronary arteries). Other health problems, like lung and kidney disease, are not uncommon. Please tell your surgeon the names of the other specialists caring for you. Your surgeon can gather information from them so that the team can make a better plan for your care before, during, and after the operation.

These surgeries take a few hours. Plan on spending one night in the ICU for observation. Typically, we use a general anesthetic. You can expect to have two large IV's and/or a central line. Also expect an arterial line in the wrist. It is important to be able to follow the blood pressure closely when we work on blood vessels. Also, IV access is important in the event that you need to urgently receive IV fluid or blood. If you have religious or personal preferences regarding blood, please make that clear to the anesthesiologist, surgeon, nurses, and staff.

A-V (arteriovenous) fistulas and grafts are other types of blood vessel surgery. The fistulas or grafts are used for dialysis in patients with kidney failure. Typically, these are placed in either arm. Many times, patients will have a general anesthetic, but appropriately-selected patients can have a MAC anesthetic. Patients undergoing dialysis usually have a number of medical problems. Additionally, placing an IV, including a central line, is often difficult. Careful discussion with your anesthesiologist will determine which type of anesthetic is most appropriate for you.

Brain

Certain, but not many, procedures can be done with simple sedation. If this option is available, it may be preferred to avoid some unwanted effects of a general anesthetic on blood flow to the brain. Perhaps the procedure will be very quick. Perhaps the surgeon will need to communicate with you to assure he is working on the correct part of the brain. Not to worry. You are given enough medication that you won't be bothered. It sounds a lot worse than it is.

More often, a general anesthetic is used for brain surgery. Since it is important for us to stay on top of the blood pressure, we generally place an arterial line in the wrist. It allows us to monitor the blood pressure with every heart beat. You can also expect a second IV. Happily, brain surgery typically isn't very painful. However, since your surgeon will want to assess your mental status in the recovery room, you may not be given any 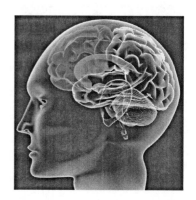 sedation before the procedure starts. That's OK. We don't want anything clouding an accurate assessment of how you're doing after surgery. With or without sedation before surgery, know that everyone is focused on making you safe and comfortable.

Breast

The breast is a very intimate part of the woman's body, and so there is often significant fear about breast surgery. With respect to the anesthesia, the most common approach is a general anesthetic. Unless the surgery is very simple and very near the surface of the breast, the surgery is often too stimulating to only have sedation (MAC). Interestingly, the pain *following* most breast surgeries isn't very severe. The exception is a breast augmentation.

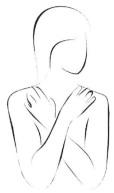

Regarding the anesthesia, the greatest risk is nausea. This is particularly true if you have a history of motion sickness. There are several medications to minimize this risk, and you can certainly request some or all of them. Pain medicines can cause nausea as well. Taking your pain pills with food and with an anti-nausea medicine may help make your recovery more pleasant.

There are some fancy ways to modify the anesthesia, and you may be offered some of these options for a breast procedure. Since a general anesthetic carries the risk of nausea, some anesthesiologists offer the combination of sedation (MAC) along with a nerve block or epidural. Like our other blocks, this block is placed under sedation, so you are not bothered by it. The thoracic (middle of the back) epidural is similar to the epidural used in pregnancy except that it's placed higher in the back. Should you be offered either of these, they are reasonable to consider, particularly if you have a high tolerance to pain medicine or a low tolerance to pain.

Children

Children are a unique class because they have unique physiology. A child is not just a smaller version of an adult. Most pediatric procedures are quick, but in this short time, complications can occur. Those complications are rare. The discussion of anesthetics for neonates and infants (less than one year) or for children with significant medical problems is beyond the scope of this text.

In some institutions, a parent is allowed to go into the OR with the child to observe the induction of anesthesia. I do not recommend this. Many children can be distracted with toys and stories about favorite movies. Some kids never even cry. Parents, however, get gripped by fear, and the children can sense it. So, an otherwise distracted, calm child gets upset because he senses that his parent is nervous/unsettled/frightened. A crying child then has to be restrained, which makes the crying worse and furthers a parent's distress. A vicious, unhelpful cycle begins. Moreover, the anesthesiologist then has to appease both the parent and the child. I recommend to parents that both they and their child will be better off *if only* the child and the anesthesiologist go into the OR.

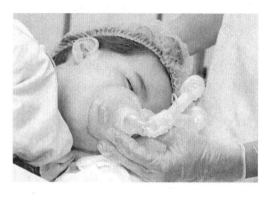

Once in the operating room, monitors are placed. This is a good time to play age-appropriate games. The monitors beep, and colors light up. We provide sleeping medicine via a mask. For children, a general anesthetic is the common choice. We start with some nitrous oxide (laughing gas), and we add in the more potent anesthesia gas. As the anesthesia deepens, the child can become hyperactive (arms and legs may move or the child may cry). As you might imagine, this could be distressing for a parent who wouldn't know to expect it. It is normal. The anesthetic continues to be deepened, and the child goes off to sleep. At this point, the IV is placed, and it is generally wrapped up in an Ace bandage so that the he or she won't pull it out easily after surgery. It's easier for us to place after the child is asleep because children usually don't sit still for a needle stick. After the IV, a breathing tube of some type may be placed. Sometimes, we can keep the child asleep by holding the breathing mask in place instead of inserting a tube.

At the conclusion of the surgery, we let the child "breathe off" the anesthesia gas. He will slowly wake up, and we usually provide blow-by oxygen next to his mouth. Parents are generally brought into the recovery room soon after surgery, because the comfort of a parent is far more effective than IV medications, even IV pain medications. Children will cry when waking up, even when there is no pain. At this point, we see that the parents were oftentimes more distressed than their child! We understand. Hug him. Hold her. Now that you're there, they'll be fine...and so will you.

Colonoscopy

A colonoscopy (co-lun-OSS-co-pee) involves the use of a lighted, flexible scope that passes through the anus into the rectum and the colon. Many times, this procedure is done as a screening for colon cancer. It is often recommended at the age of 50, but there may be reasons to have it before then. The procedure generally doesn't take long, but the prep (fluid you must drink) the night before can be unpleasant. You will spend much of the day in the bathroom. Don't plan to have guests over that night! It is important to drink all of the prep so that what comes out is mostly clear. Otherwise, the gastroenterologist won't be able to see much. And then you have to repeat the process.

In the diagram, the colon is the larger section of bowel that wraps around the abdomen. Note that the image is drawn as if you were looking at someone else. Following the picture, the procedure begins in the rectum, moves to the right and over the top and down into the left side toward the cecum, where you can see the small appendix.

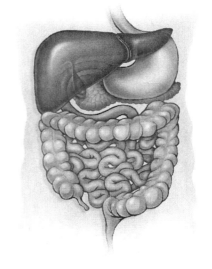

You will receive MAC anesthesia. Unless there are serious health issues in play, propofol is the drug of choice. Generally, no medication is given until the procedure is ready to begin. The propofol quickly puts you off to sleep, and you wake up within minutes of the procedure's completion. You will be asked to pass gas before you leave, so please don't be embarrassed by that. It's necessary. If it helps, know that I used to work with a nurse whose name was Tootie!

CT (CAT) Scan and MRI

These are diagnostic studies and are not surgery. However, some procedures are done with CT-guidance (a liver biopsy, for example). Even if there is no procedure involved, some patients have a hard time enduring the test. The loud noises of the machines compound an underlying claustrophobia. The fact that the test can take half an hour or more and that you must lie on an uncomfortable surface only makes things worse. The vast majority of patients tolerate the scans just fine. For those who cannot, there are some options. Nurses, under the order of a physician, can administer small amounts of sedation. For patients whose bodies are accustomed to pain medicine or relaxing medicine, higher levels of medication are required. This is also the case for patients who may have back problems or an extreme fear of the procedure. Children may also need sedation.

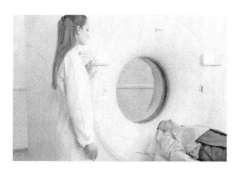

If a more aggressive approach is needed, anesthesiologists get involved. We can provide higher doses of the usual sedation, and we can also add propofol if necessary. In these cases, we will be in the control room, not in the exam room with you. That is because all people, including us, should be exposed to the least amount of radiation possible. You will be monitored, but we are separated by a small distance. As such, we are very vigilant to assure that your vital signs remain stable. We do not want to over-sedate you. Plan to be in a state of comfort and relaxation, not unconsciousness. Recall from our earlier discussion of MAC anesthesia that you can be awake and have no memory of the event. That would be ideal here.

Ear

There are three parts to the ear: outer, middle, and inner...a very intuitive naming system! The outer ear is what your mom thumped when you were talking in church. The middle ear is where the eardrum is located, as well three important little bones (incus, malleus, and stapes, pronounced EENK-us, MAL-e-us, and STAY-peez). The inner ear is near the brain and contains the cochlea, which is responsible for hearing, and a system that guides your balance. Depending on where the surgery is occurring, the anesthetic for procedures on the ear can vary wildly.

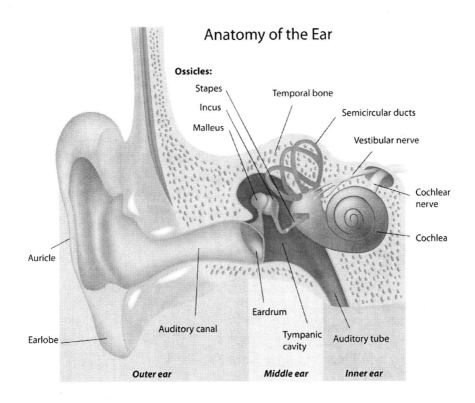

Anatomy of the Ear

Outer ear procedures are fairly simple, so the anesthesia is often MAC. A little sedation will take care of you while you have your lump, bump, or mole removed. When we move into the middle ear, a general anesthetic is necessary. The most important reason for using a general anesthetic is that you simply cannot move during this delicate surgery. Eardrum repairs or pediatric ear tubes fall into this category. When we move into the inner ear, we start thinking in terms similar to brain surgery. This surgery is extremely delicate, and a general anesthetic is mandatory. No other special anesthetic considerations are needed, except what may be required due to underlying patient issues.

There is a higher than average incidence of nausea with a general anesthetic and ear surgery. If you have a problem with nausea, particularly motion sickness, alert your anesthesiologist to this. He will provide a number of medications before and during your procedure to minimize this risk.

Endoscopy

An endoscopy (en-DOSS-co-pee) is also called an EGD. It involves the use of a lighted, flexible scope to go down the mouth, through the esophagus, and into the stomach. It also passes into the first part of the small intestine (the duodenum). In the diagram, the esophagus is at the very top, and it empties into the stomach. Understand that the image is drawn as if you were looking at someone else. The stomach is next to the liver. Careful inspection will show the duodenum exiting the stomach behind the liver. This procedure is for patients who are having abdominal pain, nausea and vomiting, severe gastric reflux, Barrett's esophagus, or even in those who may have a stuck piece of chicken!

We use MAC anesthesia for this type of procedure, which is often very quick. Propofol is the mostly commonly used drug, and oftentimes you will receive no sedation until the procedure is about to start. The propofol is given, and you wake up a few minutes later. Since the drug wears off so quickly, you leave the facility feeling wide awake and just fine. Since we are going down the same hole through which you breathe (the mouth!), there is a risk of impaired breathing or aspiration. Significant issues are 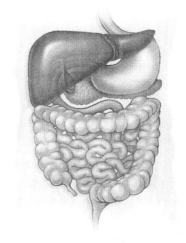 rare, and your anesthesiologist can discuss with you whether he feels these are major concerns in your care. If they are, he may suggest the use of ketamine, a drug that was discussed earlier.

Nausea is uncommon with propofol, but the physical, mechanical manipulation of your GI tract by the camera can cause nausea. Still, this is rare. Also, you may have a bit of a sore throat from the procedure, but this is also uncommon. In the vast majority of cases, there are no anesthesia problems.

Eye

As with the ear, anesthesia for the eye can vary considerably. When I had laser vision surgery, I had no anesthesia. For cataract removal, you will have some numbing drops and some light IV sedation. Simple cosmetic surgeries can be done with MAC. If you were to have eye muscle surgery or another invasive procedure, then you would have a general anesthetic. For problems that extend back behind the globe of the eye, consultation with a neurosurgeon is common, and the considerations for brain surgery apply. The vast majority of eye 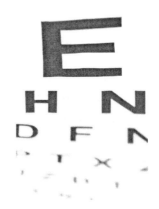 surgeries do not require anything more than some light IV sedation. As with the ear, eye surgeries carry a higher than average risk of nausea with a general anesthetic. If you have a history of nausea, particularly with motion sickness, please tell your anesthesiologist.

Face

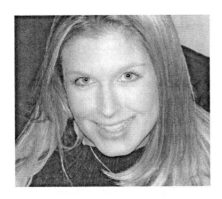 The degree of anesthesia varies depending upon the degree of surgical stimulation. For lump, bump, and mole removal, MAC sedation is often all that is necessary. For patients having major cosmetic or reconstructive procedures, general anesthesia is required. The greatest issue here is the airway. When the surgeon is working, the area is sterilized, and the anesthesiologist cannot touch it without

disrupting the surgery. Therefore, it is important that the airway be secured at the beginning of the surgery so that it is not compromised at any point during the procedure. This is typically accomplished with a breathing tube.

Also, head / neck surgery is associated with a higher incidence of nausea post-operatively. Again, if you have a history of nausea after surgery or a problem with motion sickness, it is important that you tell your anesthesiologist. There are some medications that can reduce this side effect.

Foot (podiatry)

For foot surgeries, the anesthesia is oftentimes MAC. The podiatrist will numb the foot after you have been given some sedation. In this case, you would not likely remember the procedure and you would not have a breathing tube. A general anesthetic with a breathing tube is also common, 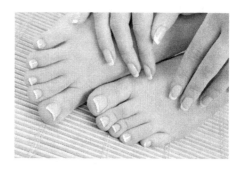 based on your preference and any medical issues you may have. As an example, patients who have severe sleep apnea or who are morbidly obese may do better with a breathing tube. A spinal is an option, but it is probably unnecessary, as the spinal lasts 2 hours longer than most foot surgeries. Waiting in the recovery room for your legs to wake up can be both boring and distressing, particularly when you're wide awake and hungry!

Gall bladder

The gall bladder is shaped like a bulb. It is under the liver, which is on the right side of the abdomen. In the diagram, it is the structure mostly hidden by the liver. The image is drawn as if you were looking at someone else, which is why it is on the left side of the picture.

Reasons for removing the gall bladder include inflammation, presence of stones, or failure to function. Your surgeon can explain further. The most common surgical approach is laparoscopic (using cameras). Several small holes are made, and they usually close nicely. There is not a tremendous amount of pain involved, and most patients go home the next day. The alternative approach is to open the abdomen. Some patients will need this because they have had multiple abdominal surgeries or perhaps because the laparoscopic attempt is too difficult.

For the surgery, plan to have a general anesthetic. We will place a breathing tube after you go to sleep. Other considerations during abdominal surgery are function of your underlying medical problems. For example, a patient who has been vomiting for two days will likely have an electrolyte imbalance and dehydration, which will require an additional large IV for rehydration. A patient with gall bladder cancer may need a central line for IV nutrition after surgery. A very sick 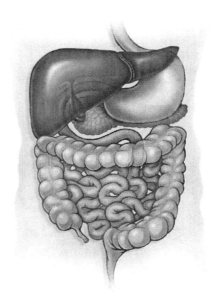 patient may need an arterial line to monitor changes in blood pressure. Patients with a difficult airway might require special equipment for placing a breathing tube. Your anesthesiologist will discuss this with you. There are too many possibilities to list here, but the ones just mentioned are common considerations.

Nausea is possible after abdominal surgery. If you have a history of motion sickness or nausea during a previous surgery, please let your anesthesiologist know. He can provide several medications to minimize this risk.

Hand

Much of the information in Arm and Forearm applies here. But, unlike the arm and forearm, many cases in the hand involve just soft tissue, and are therefore less painful after surgery. A carpal tunnel release is a good example. In this case, there is no need for a 12-18 hour nerve block. For this type of surgery, you can have MAC, a general, or a short-acting nerve block. One short-acting nerve block is called a Bier (not "beer", but pronounced the same way) block. It effectively numbs the wrist and hand for 20-30 minutes, allows you to receive simple sedation, and provides complete return of feeling at the conclusion of the case. It is useful for short cases that have fairly strong surgical stimulation but little pain afterward.

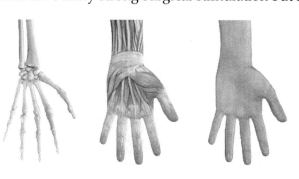

For more complicated surgeries or for cases involving bones, the regional nerve block remains an excellent choice, either by itself or in conjunction with MAC or a general anesthetic. The nerve block can be the 12-18 hour kind that completely numbs the arm, or it can be the 2-4 hour kind that numbs a particular part of the wrist or finger. Again, none of this will be done without your consent, and you do not need to feel forced into accepting this approach. If you choose to avoid a nerve block, that is fine. We will simply induce a general anesthetic (or MAC if we can) and give you the necessary IV pain medicines to keep you comfortable.

Heart, angiogram/angioplasty/ablation

The sedation for an angiogram or an angioplasty (placing a stent) may not require an anesthetic. The procedure is essentially painless, except for a small incision in the groin (which has been numbed). The registered nurses in the room typically provide IV sedation in small amounts. Patients who are very tolerant to medications or who are unable to lie still may require an anesthesia provider. For them, we use some of our more powerful drugs.

An ablation is done for an irregular heart beat, such as atrial fibrillation (a-fib). The procedure requires several hours, and so anesthesiologists are more often involved. Some anesthesiologists prefer MAC, while others prefer a general anesthetic. You and your anesthesiologist will determine what is best for you, based on your preferences and medical history. There is minimal surgical discomfort after the procedure, but you may have to lie down for several hours with pressure over your groin incision. This is to prevent bleeding out of the small incision.

Heart, open heart

Two common cases in this category include heart bypass (CABG, pronounced "cabbage", which is coronary artery bypass grafting) and valve replacement surgeries. It is "open heart" because the breastbone is opened, revealing the chest cavity. There is considerable workup that is done prior to surgery. Your anesthesiologist will review the results with you and discuss any issues of concern. You can expect to have an arterial line in a wrist, a large IV in both hands, and/or a central line. After one IV is in, you typically get some sedation before the other lines are placed.

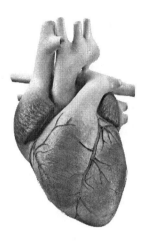

Surprisingly, the breastbone typically isn't very sore after this surgery. Expect to be the ICU for a day or two after the procedure. You will have some drains in the chest, which will come out as indicated during the course of your stay. It is becoming increasingly common to have a fast wake-up from open heart surgery. You should be be getting out of bed soon. It is important to get up and around, as activity will reduce the chance of your developing pneumonia.

Hernias (inguinal, umbilical, and abdominal)

A hernia occurs when something pokes through a wall that normally contains it. This is usually seen somewhere on the belly (abdomen). An inguinal (EENG-win-uhl) hernia is a groin hernia. An umbilical (um-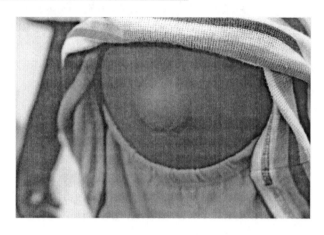
BILL-e-cull) hernia is a hernia of the belly button, which is shown in the photo. An abdominal hernia occurs somewhere else on the belly.

Depending on surgeon preference and patient issues, an inguinal hernia can be done under a general anesthetic or a MAC. This is the case if the hernia is repaired in the open fashion. Some patients prefer to be "all the way" to sleep, while others may like the idea of sedation. Both are acceptable in the proper patient and with an agreeable surgeon. If the surgeon prefers a laparoscopic approach for the inguinal hernia, then a general anesthetic is necessary.

For umbilical and abdominal hernias, a general anesthetic is required. Whether an open or laparoscopic approach is chosen, the patient needs to be all the way to sleep. The surgeries don't take very long, and the discomfort is typically mild.

Nausea is possible after abdominal surgery. If you have a history of motion sickness or nausea during a previous surgery, please let your anesthesiologist know. He can provide several medications to minimize this risk.

Hip pinning (for a fracture)

This procedure is done for a broken hip, and it is a quicker procedure than a total hip replacement (see below). A general anesthetic is often the choice here. We may avoid a spinal block in this situation for several reasons. First, many anesthesiologists perform spinal blocks with the patient sitting. This would be painful for a patient with 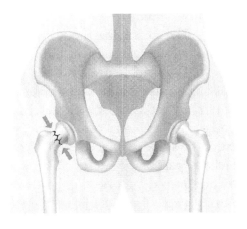 a broken hip. Second, it could displace the fracture, making the procedure more difficult for the surgeon. Third, hip fractures occur in older patients, who are often taking blood thinners for other medical problems. If this is the case, it is unsafe to perform a spinal block. Still, in the appropriate patient, a spinal block can be an excellent choice. Your anesthesiologist will explain what he thinks is best for you.

Also, be aware that while this is not typically an emergency case, it is an urgent case. That means that we may not need to perform the surgery immediately, but we ought to do it in the next day or two. Your other health problems may not be as optimized as they could be. This increases the risk of problems both during and after the surgery, despite the chosen anesthetic. There may not be much that can be done about this, but you should discuss your concerns with your anesthesiologist.

Hip replacement

A hip replacement is an elective procedure. This is not done for a broken hip, but rather for arthritis of the joint. As such, we have a few more options for the anesthesia. Typically, a general or spinal anesthetic is reasonable.

For a general anesthetic, you are completely asleep during the procedure, and you later wake up with the ability to move the legs. You will likely be braced so that you don't move your hip, however. There is a slight risk of nausea associated with a general anesthetic, but medications can significantly reduce that risk. Pain typically is mild.

The spinal anesthetic numbs the body from the belly button down. The spinal anesthetic is a nice option because it allows you to be minimally sedated (or moderately, if you prefer) and very comfortable. After the spinal is placed, you do not feel any part of the surgery. Pain medications do not need to be given during a spinal anesthetic because the body has zero sensation where the spinal is working. However, the drug commonly used in spinals will last approximately 3 hours. You may find that your waiting in the recovery room, during which time you cannot move your legs or eat anything, to be both boring and distressing. Still, in some patients it is a good (and even preferred) option.

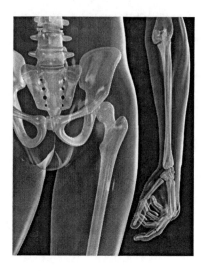

Intestine (bowel)

The bowel is another word for intestine. The intestine is made up of the small intestine (duodenum, jejunum, and ileum are its three parts) and the large intestine (colon). Sometimes, part of the bowel is removed due to an obstruction, which is oftentimes an emergency, or for a tumor. There are other reasons to operate on the intestine, as well. There are two surgical approaches: laparoscopic (using cameras) and open. For the laparoscopic approach, several small holes are made, and they usually close nicely. In the open approach, an incision is made, straight up and down, in the middle of the belly. Your surgeon will tell you which approach he thinks is most appropriate for you.

For the surgery, plan to have a general anesthetic. You may have a tube placed in the nose that goes back into the throat and down into the stomach. It is called an NG tube (NasoGastric, meaning nose-to-stomach). The tube is connected to suction so that it can constantly drain any stomach contents. In the case of an obstructed bowel, it is very important. If contents can't go *down* the bowel (like they're supposed to), then those contents come back *up!*

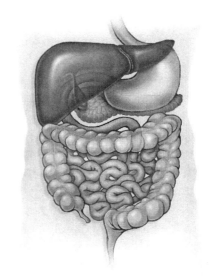

The NG tube keeps those contents sucked out of the stomach before they make it into your mouth! The tube is placed in the OR after you are asleep, but it is usually the most aggravating part of your hospital stay. It can cause a sore throat, and it is generally uncomfortable. It is very important, however. After surgery, take care not to pull it out, as it will have to be put back in...and this time, you're awake. It typically stays in about two days, and it comes out when your surgeon says so. We all know that it's unpleasant, but please understand it is for your safety.

Other considerations during abdominal surgery are functions of your underlying medical problems. For example, a patient who has been vomiting for two days will likely have an electrolyte imbalance and dehydration, which will require an additional large IV for rehydration. A patient with cancer may need a central line for IV nutrition after surgery. A very sick patient may need an arterial line to monitor changes in blood pressure. Your anesthesiologist will discuss this with you. There are several possibilities, and the ones just mentioned are common considerations.

Nausea is possible after abdominal surgery. If you have a history of motion sickness or nausea during a previous surgery, please let your anesthesiologist know. He can provide several medications to minimize this risk.

Kidney

In this section, we discuss the anesthesia for those procedures directly on the kidney. For kidney stones, please see the following section. For procedures related to the bladder, please see that section.

There are two kidneys. They are bean-shaped and located in the back of the abdomen, near the bottom of the ribs. The kidneys clear some of the body's waste and regulate fluid balance by producing urine. They kidneys drain that urine through the ureter into the bladder.

Some patients need nephrostomy (nef-ROSS-to-me) tubes to drain the kidneys. For some reason, the kidneys will not drain normally. This procedure is often done in the radiology department with some simple sedation. Some patients may require higher doses of medications or may have some other significant health problems. In this case, an anesthesiologist may get involved. Local anesthesia is applied to the skin, and live X-ray is used to guide the radiologists. With a little sedation, most patients do well.

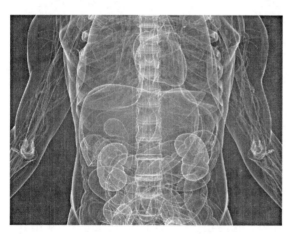

Patients who need surgery on the kidney will require a general anesthetic. The surgery can be performed to work on, remove, or transplant the kidney. Some surgeries are done open, and some use a 4-armed robot with laparoscopic cameras. Your surgeon will explain which approach is most appropriate. The nature of the surgery and your other medical problems will determine the other anesthetic considerations. Most general anesthetics for kidney surgery are very standard, even for the kidney transplant. It is reasonable, however, for very sick patients to have a central line and an arterial line.

Nausea is possible after abdominal surgery. If you have a history of motion sickness or nausea during a previous surgery, please let your anesthesiologist know. He can provide several medications to minimize this risk.

The dialysis patient does present an anesthetic challenge. Regardless of the surgical procedure (on the kidney or not), dialysis patients have more complicated issues. The dialysis process (usually 3 times per week) tends to dehydrate patients, and we cannot aggressively rehydrate them. Since there are no functioning kidneys, the body can't tolerate that. Also, these patients have been subjected to multiple needle sticks in the past. Placing an IV is very difficult. The same is often true even for central lines. Finally, dialysis patients also tend to have other significant health problems, like diabetes and heart disease. Dialysis has done a remarkable job at prolonging the lives of patients with end-stage kidney disease. However, there are multiple issues that these patients and their families should discuss with the anesthesiologist so that the planned surgical procedure goes as smoothly as possible.

Kidney stone, shock

This procedure is called an ESWL, or extracorporeal shock wave lithotripsy. ESWL is often pronounced EZZ-wall. In this procedure, no incision is made. Instead, sound waves are carefully directed at the 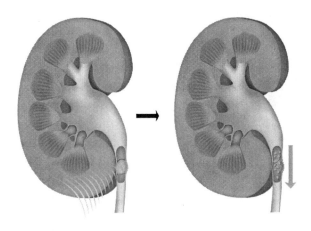 kidney stone to break it apart. In the left side of the diagram, the stone is in the light brown tube that drains the kidney. Shock waves are directed toward the stone. On the right side of the picture, the stone fragments are shown passing down the tube toward the bladder (and ultimately out of the body).

While there is no cutting, the shock waves are painful, so you can expect a general anesthetic. The procedure typically takes less than half an hour. Soreness is common, but it pales in comparison to the pain of the kidney stone. This procedure is different from a cystoscopy (see Bladder, cystoscopy), in which a camera is advanced up the urethra into the bladder to retrieve stones near the kidney. Barring other medical problems, the anesthetic for an ESWL is straightforward, and its recovery is quick.

Knee arthroscopy

A knee arthroscopy (ar-THROS-co-pee) is also called a knee scope. Two small incisions are made for the camera and instrument. It is often performed to determine the source of knee pain and/or to remove damaged structures in the knee. There are three ways this anesthetic might be administered. The most common approach is the general anesthetic. That is, you go all the way to sleep and wake up when the surgery is done. Pain medicine is given through the IV, and most patients experience only soreness after the procedure.

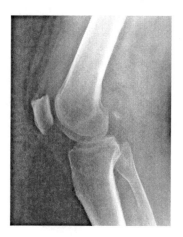

A less common approach is the spinal anesthetic. Recall that the spinal anesthetic is a single shot in the low back that will numb your body from about the belly button down. Both legs will be numb for about 3 hours. If you wish, you could have the surgery without any other medications: you could be wide awake to watch the procedure on the monitors. Most people don't care anything about this! Additionally, since the procedure only takes about 30 minutes, you will be sitting in the recovery room for a few hours while your legs wake up enough for you to bear weight and get home. Since the duration of the anesthesia and surgery don't match very closely, the spinal isn't often chosen. It can be done, however, if that is your preference.

The third, and even less common approach, is to place local anesthesia around and inside the knee, called a knee block. To this, we add MAC sedation. This is a nice approach in that you do not need the breathing tube required for a general and you do not have the numb legs of a spinal. However, the surgery needs to be completed in about 20 minutes, as the surgery itself will wash away the local anesthesia (and, therefore, the numbness). If you have a surgeon comfortable with this anesthesia, it can be an elegant approach.

Knee replacement

A knee replacement is more involved than the knee arthroscopy. An incision about 8 inches long is made over the knee. Saws and hammers are involved. The surgeon will want you moving the knee soon afterward. So it is no surprise that knee replacements can be fairly uncomfortable after surgery.

For the surgery itself, there are two options, and each of them comes with a bonus. The first option is the general anesthetic. Again, you are all the way asleep, and a breathing tube of some type is placed after the induction of anesthesia. The vital signs are monitored, and IV pain medicine, among other medications, is given according to those vital signs.

The second option is the spinal anesthetic. This is the single shot of numbing medication placed in the fluid found in the vertebral column (cerebrospinal fluid, or CSF). The numbing effect extends from the belly button to include both legs. After the spinal is placed, you can receive a little or a lot of sedation, based on your preference. The spinal lasts a little longer than the surgery, which works out well. There is little unnecessary, wasted time in the recovery room waiting for the spinal to wear off. It wears off about the time you'd be ready to go to your regular room anyway!

The "bonus" that I referenced above is called a nerve block. For many bone surgeries, we can do nerve blocks. This is a great way to lessen the requirements for general anesthesia during the surgery, as well as to make the postoperative period more comfortable. There are two major nerves in the leg. The femoral (FEM-ur-ul) nerve is in the middle of the thigh at the groin. It provides feeling to about 60% of the knee. This is an important, and, luckily, straightforward nerve to block. The sciatic (sigh-AT-ic) nerve is on the back side of the leg. It provides sensation to about 40% of the knee. If we block both nerves, the one leg becomes almost completely numb. The blocks last 12-24 hours. You can discuss this option with both your surgeon and anesthesiologist. Nerve blocks are not mandatory, and both general and spinal anesthetics are reasonable choices.

Leg, lower

Typically, this is a tibia (the larger of the two leg bones below the knee) fracture, and a rod or plate needs to be placed to align the fracture. The image depicts a tibia fracture near the ankle. A repair of an ankle fracture is another example in this category. These are very stimulating procedures, as are all bone surgeries. MAC would be unsuitable under these circumstances. The better approach would either be a general anesthetic or a spinal anesthetic.

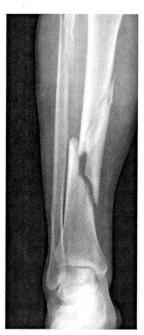

For the general anesthetic, you are completely asleep during the procedure. There is a slight risk of nausea associated with a general anesthetic, but medications can significantly reduce that risk.

The spinal anesthetic numbs the body from the belly button down. The spinal anesthetic is a nice option because it allows you to be minimally sedated (or moderately, if you prefer) and very comfortable. After the spinal is placed, you do not feel any part of the surgery. Pain medications do not need to be given during a spinal anesthetic because the body has zero sensation where the spinal is working. However, the drug commonly used in spinals will last approximately 3 hours. You may find that your waiting in the recovery room, during which time you cannot move your legs or eat anything, to be both boring and distressing. Still, in some patients it is a good (and even preferred) option.

In addition, your anesthesiologist may offer a nerve block. This is a great way to lessen the requirements for general anesthesia and pain medicine during the surgery, as well as to make the postoperative period more comfortable. There are two major nerves in the leg. The femoral (FEM-ur-ul) nerve provides feeling to the inside of the lower leg down to the bony bump at the ankle. The sciatic (sigh-AT-ic) nerve is on the back side of the leg. It provides sensation to everything else below the knee. If we block both nerves, the leg becomes almost completely numb. If we just block the sciatic nerve, we knock out most of the pain, and you can still move the upper part of the leg. The blocks last 12-24 hours. You can discuss this option with both your surgeon and anesthesiologist to determine if it makes sense for you. A nerve block is not mandatory, and both general and spinal anesthetics are reasonable choices.

Leg, upper

Surgery on the thigh is less common than surgery below the knee. A procedure here could simply be a muscle biopsy. For this, a small amount of sedation is all that is required. Alternatively, the femur bone could be fractured. In this case, considerably more anesthesia is required. Two options include a general or spinal anesthetic.

Bone surgery can be quite uncomfortable postoperatively. With a spinal anesthetic, there is no pain during surgery or for a couple of hours thereafter. Both legs are completely asleep, and the patient can have a little or a lot of sedation, based on his preference. With a general anesthetic, the patient is completely asleep, and pain medicines are given during the surgery. There is no needle stick in the back, but the leg may be a bit uncomfortable when the patient wakes up. Both are reasonable and safe in the appropriate patient. Other modifications to the anesthesia would be related to patient health issues or surgeon's needs. An example would be the need for a blood transfusion if the patient had severe trauma.

Liver

Although it doesn't always get a lot of attention, the liver is extremely important. In fact, you cannot <u>live</u> without your <u>liver</u>. The liver is a very powerful filter for drugs and toxins. It also synthesizes many enzymes and factors that the body needs. Unfortunately, major problems can occur in the liver, like cirrhosis and cancer. To better determine the cause of a problem, patients may need a liver biopsy or an even more significant procedure. In the body, the liver is on the right side of the abdomen. In the drawing, the liver is the large, wedge-shaped structure in the upper left. The image is drawn as if you were looking at someone else, which is why it is on the left side of the picture.

For a liver biopsy, which may be done with CT scan guidance, MAC is often all that is required. A little sedation relaxes the patient for the short procedure. Also, a biopsy can be a component of another procedure, like a gall bladder removal, which is done under a general anesthetic. Some patients need an even more involved procedure on the liver. In this case, plan on a general anesthetic, as the surgeon will likely want to open the abdomen. Since the liver contains so much blood, an 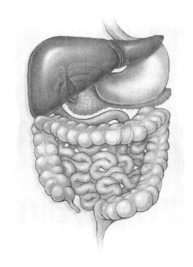 arterial line and large IV's or a central line are reasonable. There can be a lot of blood loss. For major liver operations, you should decide whether you are willing to receive a blood transfusion.

The most significant liver operation is the liver transplant. This is done in patients who have end-stage liver disease and who often have other medical problems. These patients are very sick. These are major surgeries that are usually done at large hospitals. Very large IV's are placed, at least one arterial line is placed, and multiple units of blood are administered. The surgery takes several hours. Patients should expect to stay in the ICU for several days. These are critically ill patients undergoing significant surgery with a host of physiologic changes throughout the procedure. It is very challenging for the anesthesiologist and the surgeon. Understand that the doctors who do this do it regularly, and they are the best equipped to provide the best possible outcome.

Lung

A thoracotomy (thor-a-COT-o-me) is the name of the procedure performed to remove a piece of lung, biopsy some tissue in the chest, or carry out some other related procedure. For this type of case, it is common to place an arterial line in the wrist for blood pressure monitoring and a central line for IV fluid and medication administration. Then, a general anesthetic is induced.

A thoracotomy can be uncomfortable afterward. In some institutions, the patients are offered a thoracic (middle of the back) epidural. An epidural provides excellent pain relief from the incision of a thoracotomy. Good pain relief allows for better breathing and greater 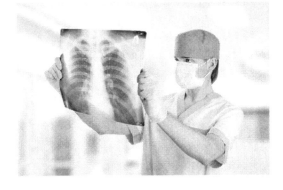 activity, both of which decrease the risk for pneumonia after surgery. While there is technically a higher risk with this epidural than with an epidural for a laboring pregnant woman (lower back), the likelihood of having a problem is very low. It is critical that you tell the anesthesiologist if you have been taking blood thinners. If you prefer to avoid the epidural, that is fine. IV pain medication is also a reasonable alternative.

Depending on the reason for the thoracotomy, it is possible that you will retain the breathing tube after surgery. If this happens, sedation is provided so that you will remain relaxed. If the tube is removed, a sore throat is not uncommon. You should also expect to stay in the ICU for the first night. Deep breathing and coughing are very important in the recovery from this surgery.

Major trauma

The purpose of this text is to provide patients with information *before* they have surgery. Obviously, this is silly when we consider major trauma. After all, who is going to read this and then plan on having a serious car accident?! Still, for the sake of completeness, let us consider some issues. In trauma, we follow the ABC's: airway, breathing, circulation. A trauma patient will almost always get a breathing tube. Then, we will breathe for him using a ventilator. We will give IV fluids, including blood if necessary, through very large IV's. An arterial line and a central line are not uncommon.

Many trauma patients need immediate surgery. Family is not allowed in the operating rooms. In the ER, things happen very fast, and they should. Specific anesthetic considerations change depending upon the nature of the surgery, the condition of the patient, 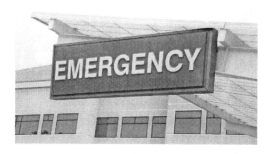 and any underlying medical conditions that may be known. Generally, the expectation should be that a breathing tube will stay in place, the patient will go to the ICU, large IV's will be placed, and lots of fluids will be given. To improve care, the family can provide the physicians with as much information as possible about those underlying medical conditions. One of the most helpful things you can do is to document your medical history (medications, allergies, medical conditions) on a small sheet of paper and put it in your wallet or purse. In case of an accident, this information helps us to take care of you much better.

Mouth

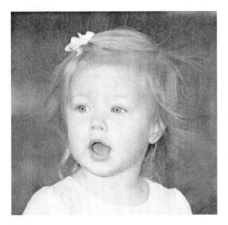

This category includes procedures like tonsillectomy, parotid gland surgery, or tongue surgery. Procedures inside the mouth typically require a general anesthetic. Surgery on the mouth can present a problem for the anesthesiologist because our biggest concern is the airway. It is our goal to make sure that you breathe and breathe well during your surgery. So we are very particular about examining your airway and talking with your surgeon about problems he may anticipate.

In patients who have a mass or other lesion in the mouth, we will often place a breathing tube via the nose. We will also do this for special-needs children who are having their teeth cleaned. This sounds unpleasant, but it is done after you are asleep. It is a better solution that inserting the tube through the mouth, which could cause bleeding that might be difficult to control. Furthermore, it may be exceedingly difficult to insert the tube, and even if we are successful, the tube just gets in the way of the surgeon who's trying to work!

After the surgery, you may find a small amount of blood in a tissue when you blow your nose. There may be some nausea associated with oral surgery, so if you have a problem with motion sickness or have a previous history of nausea after anesthesia, please tell your anesthesiologist.

Neck, bones

Neck surgery is often a last resort for patients who have suffered through pain injections, physical therapy, and daily narcotic use. Examples of neck surgeries include laminectomies and fusions. These surgeries require a general anesthetic. Before surgery, it is important that we carefully examine your airway and your neck movement. We want to know how much you can move your neck so that we don't go beyond those limitations. Please tell us if any movement is painful to you, 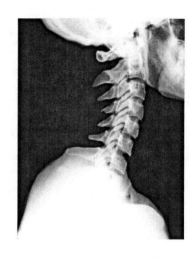 particularly if it is associated with pain down your arms. If you have a very limited range of neck motion, we may one of a variety of special tools to carefully place a breathing tube. We have a number of ways to keep you safe with respect to your airway.

If there is a significant history of narcotic use, you will require more pain medicine to be comfortable after surgery. Be very honest with your anesthesiologist about how much you are taking, as he will use that information to decide how much is the right amount for you.

Neck, carotid artery

The carotid artery is the pulse that you can feel in the side of your neck. As we get older, this artery can get clogged with plaque, which increases the risk of stroke. This can be discovered at a routine doctor visit or as a followup to your getting lightheaded when you stand up, for example. A surgeon will tell you that, at a certain point, the risk of having the procedure is lower than the risk of *not* having the procedure.

There are two anesthetics for this surgery. For either one, you can expect to have an arterial line placed in one wrist. Blood pressure monitoring is very important. To help make sure that both sides of your brain receive good blood flow, the 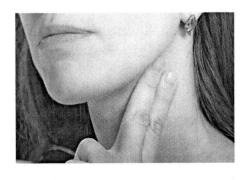 anesthesiologist will make sure that your blood pressure is appropriate. An EEG ("brain wave") technician will also monitor several small probes on your scalp to see that the neurons are working as they should.

A general anesthetic is most commonly used. In order to maintain stable blood pressure, the anesthetic is gently induced, and blood pressure is tightly controlled with IV medications that can raise and lower the pressure quickly as needed. Despite working with an artery, blood loss is typically small. Upon awakening, you will need to move your arms and legs. We want to make sure that a stroke or other problem has not occurred. The incidence of a stroke is very low, and your surgeon can provide more information about it.

The other anesthetic option is a combination of a regional anesthetic and MAC. In this instance, the anesthesiologist would perform a "deep cervical plexus block". This block is done under sedation. The local anesthesia is placed next to three vertebrae in the neck. There are lots of important structures in the neck, so the anesthesiologist will be extremely careful. After this block is placed, the surface of the skin should also be numbed. At this point, the surgery can proceed. You can be responsive to the surgeons in the OR. You can talk to them, and you can also have more sedation if you need it. Since we're working on an artery near the brain, it is important to know if the brain is getting the blood flow it needs. Your ability to talk and follow commands is a great way to know if that is the case. Some surgeons find this the best way to ensure your safety and good outcome. Understand that your ability to respond does <u>not</u> mean that you will remember the surgery or that it will be unpleasant for you.

Neck, everything else

There are many important structures in the neck, including the thyroid gland, parathyroid glands, lymph nodes, trachea (windpipe), and esophagus. Except for procedures on or just under the skin, we will induce a general anesthetic. Because there are a number of structures very close together in the neck, it is important that you don't move during the procedure. Also, as in facial surgery, gaining access to your airway is difficult due to the close proximity of the sterile neck and your mouth. So, for your safety, we will secure your airway and then get out of the surgeon's way.

Surgery on the neck can cause nausea. If you have a history of motion sickness or nausea during a previous surgery, please let your anesthesiologist know. He can provide several medications to minimize this risk.

Nose

For lumps and bumps, a MAC is more than sufficient anesthesia. The surgeon will numb the skin (local anesthesia), and your anesthesiologist will provide enough sedation to relax you. The skin here is sensitive, so extra numbing medicine and sleeping medicine are given. The wake-up is quick.

If you need surgery inside the nose and in the sinuses, a general anesthetic is necessary. Obviously, the inside of the nose is sensitive, and your surgeon won't want your moving around while he's working in there. Furthermore, you wouldn't want any chance of remembering this procedure. Understand that surgeries on the nose can be associated with nausea afterward. We treat the potential for nausea with medications. If you have a problem with motion sickness or have had nausea after surgery, please tell your anesthesiologist.

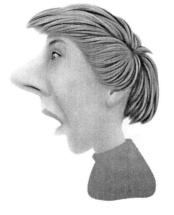

Pain injections (by your chronic pain physician)

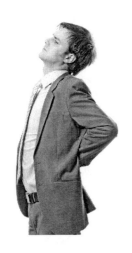

Many patients suffer from chronic pain, and they have their pain treated by a variety of injections. For the patients who have anxiety about getting the shots in the doctor's office, they can come to the OR for some sedation. These cases involve the use of MAC. Assuming there are no significant medical problems, you will get an IV, lie down on the table, and receive a little sedation. The recovery is quick, and you will be discharged with few, if any, side effects. Most people don't remember anything about the brief procedure, but know that MAC anesthesia deliberately avoids the deep sleep of a general anesthetic. Therefore, recall of sounds or lights is not worrisome. As with all anesthetics, medical conditions such as obesity, heart and lung disease, and drug tolerance make this more difficult. These are issues your anesthesiologist will discuss with you.

Prostate removal

This is called a prostatectomy (PROS-ta-TECK-to-me), and it is done to treat cancer. Oftentimes, this procedure is performed laparoscopically with the use of a 4-armed robot. It can also be done with the open approach. Your surgeon will advise you of the better approach for you. You may get two IV's. Depending on the facility's customs and your 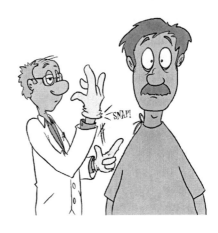 physiologic needs, you may also receive an arterial line for blood pressure monitoring.

Expect to have a urinary catheter (we call it a Foley) in place when you wake up. While it is constantly draining your bladder, you will still feel like you need to urinate. It is necessary, and it will come out as soon as possible.

Prostate seeding

A prostate seeding is done for the treatment of prostate cancer. It is an outpatient procedure that involves the strategic placement of small, radioactive "seeds" near the cancer. The anesthesia can either be MAC or general. This is determined by surgeon and patient preference, anticipated length of the procedure, and your other medical conditions. You can plan to go home afterward.

Shoulder

Rotator cuff injuries or other problems are common inside the shoulder. A general anesthetic is used, and oftentimes the repair can be done with the use of arthroscopic cameras. It sounds simple, but the pain from a shoulder operation can be intense. An anesthetic challenge is dealing with the discomfort after surgery, so it is common to suggest a nerve block.

A nerve block is discussed above under Regional Anesthesia. The appropriate block is called an interscalene (en-ter-SCAY-leen) block. This block is done on the side of the neck, halfway between the ear and collarbone, and roughly 1/2-inch deep. Sedation is provided, so the block is well-tolerated. Most people don't remember it. Depending upon 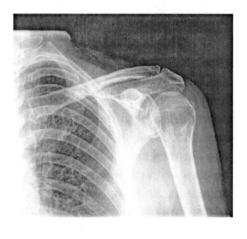 the drug injected, the block can last 12-18 hours. Indeed, you will be sore after those 12-18 hours, but consider all the pain that will have been avoided during that first day! Please understand that if you do not want a block or are not a candidate for a block, you will be given enough medicine to be as comfortable as safely possible.

Spleen

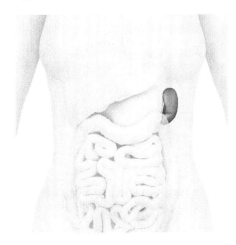

The spleen is in the upper left part of the abdomen, near the ribs. The image is drawn as if you were looking at someone else, which is why it is on the right side of the picture. Its function, among other things, is to remove old red blood cells and to eliminate some bacteria. Elective surgery on the spleen is uncommon. Most surgeries on the spleen are the result of trauma. The surgery, therefore, is to remove the spleen. This is called a splenectomy (splen-ECK-to-me).

For spleen surgery, plan on a general anesthetic. If trauma was involved, then the patient may need better IV access, including a central line, and close monitoring of the blood pressure, by way of an arterial line. Blood may need to be given. If we have no indication that the patient would refuse blood, we will give it as a lifesaving measure. Please read the sections on Major Trauma and also Blood Transfusions under Special Considerations.

Nausea is possible after abdominal surgery. While this isn't a major concern during emergency surgery, it can be something to discuss in the elective situation. If you have a history of motion sickness or nausea during a previous surgery, please let your anesthesiologist know. He can provide several medications to minimize this risk.

Uterus

A hysterectomy (HISS-ter-ECK-to-me) is the removal of the uterus. In the photo, the ovaries and Fallopian tubes are also shown. There are two common versions to this procedure: abdominal hysterectomy and vaginal hysterectomy. Your surgeon will suggest which approach he thinks is best for you. Usually, the anesthesia for either is the same: a general anesthetic. You will go all the way to sleep and wake up when the surgery is over.

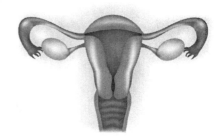

The anesthesiologist will discuss risks specific to you, but in general, women have a higher risk of nausea than men. Additionally, procedures on the sex organs carry a higher risk for nausea. If you have a problem with motion sickness or you have gotten sick after a previous anesthetic, talk with your anesthesiologist about medications to prevent nausea.

Wrist

Much of the information in Arm and Forearm applies here. But, unlike the arm and forearm, many cases in the wrist involve just soft tissue, and are therefore less painful after surgery. Removal of a ganglion cyst is a good example. In this case, there is no need for a 12-18 hour nerve block. For this type of surgery, you can have MAC, a general, or a short-acting nerve block. One short-acting nerve block is called a Bier (not "beer", but pronounced the same way) block. It effectively numbs the wrist and hand for 20-30 minutes, allows you to receive simple sedation, and provides

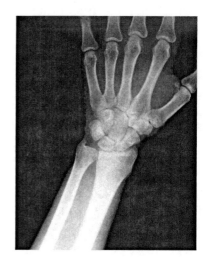

complete return of feeling at the conclusion of the case. It is useful for short cases that have fairly strong surgical stimulation but very little pain afterward.

For more complicated surgeries or for cases involving bones, the regional nerve block remains an excellent choice, either by itself or in conjunction with MAC or a general anesthetic. The nerve block can be the 12-18 hour kind that completely numbs the arm, or it can be the 2-4 hour kind that numbs a particular part of the wrist or finger. Again, none of this will be done without your consent, and you do not need to feel forced into accepting this approach. If you choose to avoid a nerve block, that is fine. We will simply induce a general anesthetic (or MAC if we can) and give you the necessary IV pain medicines to keep you comfortable.

Special Considerations

If any of these apply to you, I encourage you to carefully read the topic. Then, let your anesthesiologist know as much as you can about your history related to that matter. You will then be able to ask educated questions and participate in the designing of your anesthetic.

Allergies

A true medical allergy includes a rash, sudden drop in blood pressure, and difficulty breathing. Also understand that some medications cause a rash, and this is <u>not</u> related to an allergy. I know it's confusing, but your anesthesiologist can help you understand the difference. It is important to 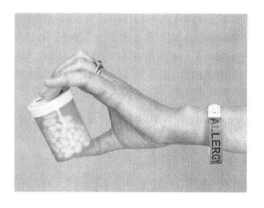 understand whether a reaction is an allergy or an unpleasant side effect. Unpleasant side effects include nausea, diarrhea, confusion, excitement, sleepiness, and the like. If you are truly allergic to a medication, then we cannot give you *anything* from that class of medications. Consider morphine. A morphine allergy is very rare, but patients tend not to like the way it makes them feel (nausea, confusion, etc.). If it were a true allergy, we could not give *any* opiate pain medications! How horrible!

Interestingly, some people say they have an allergy to Novocaine (the generic name is procaine). We hear that the allergy is a fast heart rate, and that this was discovered in the dentist's office. Is this real? No. Understand there are a lot of blood vessels under the mucosa (or skin) in the mouth. Have you ever bitten your lip? There's a lot of blood. Well, when a dentist injects the gums with Novocaine, he often uses epinephrine. Epinephrine causes the blood vessels to constrict, or tighten. This is important because it makes the Novocaine lasts longer. Here's the rub: epinephrine's other name is Adrenalin. Yes, it's what you think it is. When

Adrenalin is injected with that Novocaine...and some of it gets INSIDE the blood vessel, what do you get? An Adrenalin rush! In addition to prolonging the numbing, Adrenalin causes the heart rate to go up! Patients say they feel palpitations. They feel nervous. It's all very normal. This is not an allergy. In fact, for those readers who have severe asthma or food allergies, you know that epinephrine (Adrenalin) is a rescue *treatment* for a severe allergy!

Awareness

The topic of awareness has come up in movies and in news shows. It has been sensationalized to a degree that makes people believe the issue is far more common than it really is. Awareness is being *aware* of what is happening while under anesthesia. It is described as a patient who is thought to be sufficiently anesthetized but is aware of what is going on. *Complete, explicit* awareness is rare. Implicit awareness is limited to recall of non-specific sounds or touch. Other cases of memories after anesthesia are described as intraoperative dreaming. Studies have shown that the incidence of awareness under anesthesia ranges from around 1 in 770 to 1 in 14,700. We know there are certain patient conditions and certain surgeries in which this risk is higher, although it is possible in any kind of surgery. Anesthesiologists are very vigilant to prevent awareness. We take measures to assure that patients are unaware of the events around them during their procedures.

There are three classes of surgery during which awareness under general anesthesia is more likely, but still uncommon: trauma, cardiac, and obstetrics (Cesarean Sections). In these cases, certain factors make the usual amount of anesthesia unsafe. Care must be taken to balance safety against sleepiness.

In trauma, the patients may be bleeding severely. They have very little blood, and so their blood pressure is already low. We may not be able to give very much, if any, anesthesia gas to those patients. We recognize the risk of awareness, and so we give other medications in IV form to help. For all the trauma I did, I never knew of a patient with awareness.

In cardiac surgery, the patients are very sick. Their hearts have a hard time maintaining a good blood pressure even during a regular day at home, and this problem is made worse with our anesthetics. Again, the anesthesiologist knows this risk, and he provides medication to minimize this.

For the pregnant patient who is having a <u>general</u> anesthetic for an emergency Cesarean Section, there may be a lot of bleeding involved. Again, in patients who have a very low blood pressure already, adding a general anesthetic on top of that only aggravates the issue. Remember that most moms don't even have a general anesthetic - they have spinals! In the rare general anesthetic, we provide IV medication to minimize the risk of awareness. Again, I have never had a new mom complain of awareness!

Since dramatic blood loss and catastrophically low blood pressure are uncommon, so are the risks of awareness, particularly when all anesthesiologists are trained to be aware of the issue and treat it preemptively.

Blood transfusions and Jehovah's Witnesses

There are some 7.5 million Jehovah's witnesses, so it is not uncommon to treat these patients. In most cases, the anesthetic is in no way changed from someone who is not of that faith. From time to time, issues arise. The most common consideration is blood transfusion. It is important for the Jehovah's Witness reader (and everyone else, for that matter) to know that personal preferences *must* be expressed to the healthcare provider. You should understand that anesthesiologists do not force therapy onto patients. We respect your beliefs and will adhere to them.

From the Jehovah's Witnesses Official Media Web Site (http://www.jw-media.org/aboutjw/medical.htm), "Jehovah's Witnesses request non-blood alternatives, which are widely used and accepted by the medical community. We do this because of the Bible's command to 'keep abstaining from...blood.' [Acts 15:29]" The website continues, "Since the Bible makes no clear statement about the use of minor blood fractions or the immediate re-infusion of a

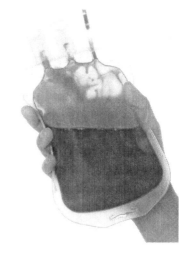

patient's own blood during surgery, a medical process known as blood salvaging, the use of such treatments is a matter of personal choice. We accept reliable non-blood medical alternatives, which are increasingly recognized in the medical field."

Before blood can be given, you must agree and sign a consent form. In an elective setting, rest assured that you will not receive any blood without your permission. The *exception to this rule* is the emergency. In an emergency, if we do not have knowledge of your preferences, we will do what we believe is medically necessary to save your life. Having some indicator of your preferences on your person will greatly increase the chances of your wishes being followed. In any case, please make clear if you will accept any of the "minor blood fractions or the immediate re-infusion of [your] blood during surgery". Patient and family communication to each and every provider is key to preventing errors, respecting personal preferences, and improving overall care.

Also understand that there are outside legal issues that must be considered when dealing with children of Jehovah's witnesses. Anesthesiologists render care as the patient wishes, but our legal system has set in place caveats under which children may get what is viewed as the more standard care. This may be unpleasant for the family, but the issues are legal ones, and, as such, fall outside the practice of medicine and also the purpose of this text.

The website above quotes Law Professor Charles H. Baron when he wrote that "patients in general enjoy greater autonomy over a whole range of health care decisions because of the work done by the Witnesses as part of an overall patients' rights movement." Indeed, all of our patients are reminded that our job is to advise you of the options, risks, and benefits, to make a recommendation, and to then do as you wish. Please help us help you by openly and honestly discussing your needs, your preferences, and your fears.

Chronic Pain

Chronic pain is difficult to treat, and it often requires the consultation of a specialist. There are multitudes of behavioral, psychological, interventional, and pharmacologic therapies to assist patients with chronic pain. For patients who take opiate pain medications, the anesthetic can be challenging. The body develops a tolerance to opiates and sedating medicines. So our pain and relaxing medications aren't typically effective at the usual doses.

When we administer our medicines, a patient with chronic pain often requires a much higher dose. When we are at your side, this is not a problem. However, we are also concerned about your welfare when you are in a regular hospital room. Will you have enough pain medicine? Because we must give large doses, will you get too much? It's a complicated issue. Your anesthesiologist may suggest some other techniques for making sure that the right amount of pain medicine is given, so that you will remain safe and comfortable.

Your anesthesiologist needs to be aware of the kinds and amounts of pain medicines that are being taken. A frank discussion about your needs and expectations is important. The anesthesiologist is there, above all, to maintain your health and safety. He will discuss a plan of medications that will provide the best pain relief possible without compromising your well-being.

Difficult Airway

Patients who breathe always do better than patients who don't! I joke with my patients about this, but there is nothing more critical to the anesthesiologist. Airway is paramount. The difficult airway is the bane of the anesthesiologist. We are the airway experts, and so we are the ones who are the last resort for the difficult airway. For the anticipated difficult airway, we simply plan ahead and use all of our tools to safely place the breathing tube, if that is what is required.

We realize that a breathing tube sounds scary. We realize that getting a breathing tube while *awake* is *really* scary. Nobody gets a breathing tube while *wide* awake. We will do everything we can to make it more pleasant. Mind you, we will do nothing to compromise your safety, but we have a surprising array of tools to address your problems. If we suspect a difficult airway, we will give you as much sedation as safely possible before we attempt to put in a tube. It's not as bad as it sounds. Feel free to discuss your concerns at any time with your anesthesiologist.

You may have a sore throat after surgery, and, if you do, it usually lasts no more than 24 hours. If you have ever been told that you have a difficult airway, please tell your anesthesiologist. It will improve your care and safety if you do.

Difficult IV Stick

In addition to being airway experts, we are also IV experts. I may not be able to get blood out of a turnip, but I can get it out of you! In many ways, someone's "bad veins" are a problem of my own making. After all, I won't let you eat or drink anything!

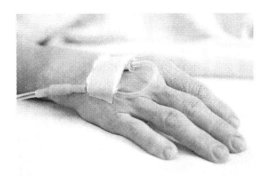

Except in some pediatric cases, an IV is a requirement for surgery. But some patients just don't have a good selection of veins. Common reasons for being a difficult IV stick include obesity, IV drug abuse, chemotherapy, multiple recent blood draws, and certain skin conditions. There is little that can be done to make a person with bad veins into a person with good veins. However, there are some intelligent ways to make the most of what veins you do have.

First, don't allow someone to stick you more than twice. Once a hole is made in a vein, that spot is useless for a day until the vein heals. If someone sticks every detectable vein...and misses...where I am going to try? Second, if you know that you're likely to be a difficult stick, don't let anyone but an anesthesiologist try. Most nurses don't care if you ask them not to poke you. It's your body. I certainly wouldn't want to endure multiple IV attempts. Third, you may only have *one good vein*. Before surgery, you may need lab work drawn. If the lab tech pokes a hole in that one good vein *before* surgery, then what am I going to use *for* the surgery?

If you think you are doing to be a difficult stick, ask to talk with the anesthesiologist. Perhaps the lab work doesn't need to be drawn or maybe it can be drawn the day of surgery *through* your IV.

Maybe you should just get a central line without enduring multiple, failed attempts. Or maybe the anesthesiologist would like to be the first one to try. In any case, be proactive in your care. In this scenario, it quite literally will be a less painful experience.

DNR (Do Not Resuscitate), Living Will, and POA

Most people like to have control over many (if not all) aspects of their life. As we get older, we begin dealing with the inevitability of death. It is increasingly common for people to make decisions regarding the degree to which lifesaving interventions are to be used. A Living Will outlines a patient's expectations for use of a feeding tube, CPR (chest compressions), rescue drugs, electrical shocks to the heart, and placement of a breathing tube. A patient's DNR states that one or more of those interventions will _not_ be used in the event of sudden cardiac arrest. A POA (Power of Attorney) designates a person who is legally authorized to make healthcare decisions for someone who is otherwise incapacitated.

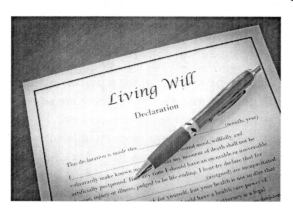

Understand that the DNR is suspended in the operating room. If the heart stops, we will intervene with all of the tools available to us. Why? There is a difference between a patient's sudden cardiac arrest while watching TV and his sudden cardiac arrest while he's receiving anesthesia and surgery. If we're giving anesthetics and performing surgery, then we are obligated to treat the complications related to those. Also, understand that if there is any confusion related to the DNR, we will always err on the side of life. It is better to try to save a life than to mistakenly allow a death.

The Living Will, DNR, and POA (when the time is right) need to be made clear. Having them takes terribly difficult decisions out of the hands of your family. It removes guesswork from the family and from the physicians. Clarity on the issue allows us to focus on the care that is needed and the way it is to be delivered.

Heart valve problems

There are four heart valves. Those valves can either be normal, too tight, or too floppy. If the valves are abnormal in any way, that can cause blood to back up into the body (or the lungs specifically), or the valves could cause the heart to become dilated or too thick. None of those conditions are ideal, and they affect the anesthesia.

A study of heart valves is unnecessary, but there are some conditions under which certain anesthetics can be problematic. The worst offender is a condition called aortic (ay-OR-tic) stenosis, a condition in which the aortic valve is too tight. If you have a valve problem, it is important that you tell your anesthesiologist, and, if you have it, bring information from your cardiologist.

Some patients have mitral (MY-trul) valve prolapse. If you have this condition, you may be accustomed to getting antibiotics before dental procedures. Mitral valve prolapse won't affect the anesthesia, but we would like to give you any necessary antibiotics to prevent you from getting an infected valve. Please tell us if you have mitral valve prolapse or any other heart valve problem.

Language challenges

¿Me entiendes? Es ist wichtig. Que devez-vous? Я хочу вам помочь. The United States is a melting pot of cultures and languages. A discussion of who should speak what language is beyond the purpose of this text, but the need for patients to be able to be understood is obvious. I had a Spanish patient who was unable to convey to his English-speaking nurse that his IV had infiltrated and was causing pain. So, his arm became swollen with fluid. This resolved without incident, but it shouldn't happen.

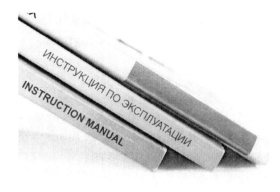

I have taken care of people who speak Spanish, French, German, Korean, Chinese, or Russian, among others. It's the nature of the country in which we live. It is *everyone's* obligation to participate in the communication process.

First, hospitals usually provide translation services for any spoken language, even if the translation occurs over the phone (as it might for lesser-encountered languages). Doctors, nurses, and staff often are bilingual, particularly in certain regions of the country. Second, it is also the patient's responsibility to do what he can to be understood. At a minimum, body language can often convey an idea even if there are no words that can be used. There is no reason that a patient should be unclean or sit in pain because he does not speak the primary language.

A language barrier isn't always English to Spanish or French to German, for example. We also take care of deaf patients who understand English...but it's by way of *American sign language*. The same rules apply here. Hospitals usually provide interpreters. Doctors and nurses are perfectly happy to speak slowly (for those lip-readers) or write down their thoughts. Patients should know that their interpreters are welcomed to join them. We will do whatever we can to allow the free flow of ideas to occur, regardless of the nature of language barrier.

Malignant Hyperthermia

If you know you have it, tell us. If you've never heard of it, you'll probably be fine. Malignant hyperthermia is the only truly life-threatening complication directly caused by some of our anesthesia medicines. There are alternative routes we can take in patients in whom we suspect have the susceptibility. In malignant hyperthermia, the anesthesia causes muscle cells to release calcium and heat up. The condition is rare and its treatment is known, but it can still be fatal. Note that this information should in no way discourage you from having surgery and anesthesia. In fact, most anesthesiologists have never seen a case of malignant hyperthermia. However, if you or a family member have this condition, please tell us.

Nausea

Patients would rather have pain than nausea. At first blush, that sounds silly. But talk to any patient who was nauseated after surgery and the story will be confirmed. So anesthesiologists make a conscientious effort to eliminate nausea after a procedure. Certain patients and certain surgeries have higher risks. Women, non-smokers, and people who have motion sickness have the highest risks. Laparoscopic (cameras in the belly) surgeries and also surgeries on the reproductive organs, breasts, and head/neck area tend to cause more nausea.

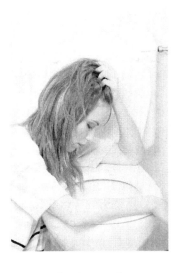

There are a number of cellular receptors in the brain that have been linked to nausea. Fortunately, we have a variety of medications that can affect those receptors, resulting in a lower likelihood of problems. Some medicines should be given early, and some are most effective when administered at the conclusion of the surgery. If you have a concern about nausea, discuss it with your anesthesiologist. In my hospital, we have a "no ralph-ing" policy!

Post-op ventilation

This means that the breathing tube is left in place after surgery. For the most part, we know before surgery who is going to have a tube after surgery. If your anesthesiologist doesn't mention it to you, don't expect that you will require one. If you come to the OR with a tube in place, we typically leave it in. If you are very sick but don't yet have a breathing tube, we will likely leave in what we put in.

Occasionally, patients will be very sensitive to our muscle relaxants or to the anesthesia itself, and the tube may be left in place temporarily. And sometimes unforeseen complications will arise that necessitate your remaining intubated (IN-too-BAY-ted). In any case, sedation will be provided so that the experience won't be as frightening as it sounds. As the doctors determine that you are ready to have the tube removed, they will lighten the sedation so that you become more responsive. As you do, your breathing will improve even more, and the tube will come out soon thereafter.

Pseudocholinesterase Deficiency

This is right up there with malignant hyperthermia. If you know you have it, tell us. If you've never heard of it, you'll probably be fine. This condition is a rare deficiency of an enzyme that is used to break down one of our muscle relaxant (paralytic) drugs. That drug is succinylcholine (SUX-e-nil-KO-leen), often just called "sux". Normally, the drug lasts about 5 minutes. With this deficiency, the drug can last an hour or more.

Even if you have the deficiency, you may not receive the drug anyway, as it's not used for everyone. Also, if the surgery lasts longer than the prolonged duration of the drug, there is no problem. If you do get the drug and its effects outlast the surgery, you will just need a breathing tube (with sedation) until the drug wears off. There are no other complications. You should be provided with information about your condition, and you may be asked to get a test called a "dibucaine (DI-byu-cane) number", which helps us know the severity of the condition. Outside of avoiding the drug, there are no other issues at stake.

An Anesthesiologist *Is* a Medical Doctor

To become an M.D., a medical doctor, one typically goes to four years of college and then four years of medical school. There are a few combined programs that offer six years to a medical degree straight after high school. After medical school, the graduate is called "doctor", but there's little that he can do in medicine. A residency is required to become whatever "type" of doctor one wants to be.

The residency could be in family practice, internal medicine, anesthesiology, general surgery, ophthalmology, or radiology, among others. As a holdover from years past (when only one year of post-graduate training was required), the first year of residency is called the internship. Subsequent years are called the residency (or some people just call the entire term a residency). If the doctor chooses to specialize even further, that training is called a fellowship. As an example, an internal medicine resident could do a fellowship in cardiology, and then another fellowship in interventional cardiology, and still another in electrophysiology. An anesthesiology resident could do a fellowship in pediatric anesthesiology.

The shortest residency is three years: family medicine, emergency medicine, and internal medicine are examples. Others are four years, like anesthesiology, OB/GYN, and ophthalmology. General surgery and urology are typically five years, and neurosurgery can be six years. So, it takes a minimum of 11 years after high school (in the traditional schools) to become a practicing physician (4 years of college + 4 years of medical school + 3 years of residency). Obviously, the obligation is longer as the residencies pass beyond three years. An anesthesiologist is a medical doctor, and the training after high school is a minimum of 12 years.

Also, understand that podiatrists, chiropractors, dentists, pharmacists, and optometrists are not medical doctors (MD's). They are doctors of podiatry (DPM), doctors of chiropractic (DC), doctors of dental surgery (DDS or DMD), doctors of pharmacy (PharmD), and doctors of optometry (OD). Their training is shorter and differently-focused. While they provide a valuable function in their specific area of training, their role is different than that of a medical doctor.

About Other People Who Administer Anesthesia

In addition to physicians, there are mid-level practitioners in many fields of medicine. Mid-level practitioners include physician assistants (PA's), advanced registered nurse practitioners (ARNP's), anesthesiologist assistants (AA's), and certified registered nurse anesthetists (CRNA's). These providers are trained in their specific areas and may, in fact, be quite skilled, but they should not be confused for physicians. Their training, by comparison, is abbreviated, and, as such, they generally do not have the knowledge or experience of a medical doctor. As a patient, you should be certain of the credentials of the people who are caring for you.

Specific to anesthesiology, we have two mid-level providers: the anesthesiologist assistant (AA) and the certified registered nurse anesthetist (CRNA). The anesthesiologist assistant can have a bachelor's degree in any field. He then attends Anesthesiologist Assistant school for two years. Conversely, a CRNA has a bachelor's degree in nursing and at least 1 year of ICU nursing experience. He then attends a two-year CRNA program. Once out of school, they both work in conjunction with the supervising anesthesiologist to administer the designed anesthetic.

Several states have opted out of the physician supervision requirement for CRNA's. This allows them to work completely free of an anesthesiologist, if a hospital or other facility is willing. The author does not support this. Consider how few of us would want a well-trained nurse to perform an operation! We would demand a well-trained surgeon! Certainly, the medical practice of anesthesiology is just as complex as the medical practice of surgery.

There are political forces that suggest that nurses are as competent as doctors in designing smooth, physiologic anesthetics. They are not; it is not in their education or training to do so. There is nothing wrong with nursing, but nurses are not medical doctors. Nurse anesthetists should not be designing anesthetics, which requires a deep understanding of physiologic and pharmacologic intricacies and subtleties, any more than their nurse practitioner counterparts should evaluate and treat complex situations like an intracranial aneurysm or septic shock. An anesthetic may seem straightforward, but it may actually be, or certainly become, very complex. I would ask for an anesthesiologist to make that assessment. After all, we are talking about your ultimate safety. Allowing a nurse anesthetist to step outside the boundaries of his nursing education, training, and role and into the education, training, and role of a physician is ill-advised.

Properly done in a team approach, with the anesthesiologist as team leader and the AA/CRNA working under his supervision, anesthetics can be rendered safely, elegantly, and efficiently. When each member performs his duties within his role, the patient's care is optimized. I think you'll find that it intuitively makes sense.

Understand that anesthesiologists' motto is "vigilance", and our focus is safety. We will work very hard to assure that you are protected, stable, and comfortable before, during, and after your procedure.

Conclusion

The administration of an anesthetic is a lot of fun. It's instant gratification. We use powerful drugs and some fantastic equipment. In real-time, we maintain a complex physiology while the surgeons rearrange the anatomy. We act quickly and decisively. It's great for us...

...and it's crazy scary for you.

Patients are often more afraid of the anesthetic than they are of the surgery. We are an unfamiliar face first seen at a very stressful time. We offer options that may sound unpleasant, and we expect you to make an immediate decision about something you don't entirely understand. You have to turn complete control over to a stranger. You wonder if you'll be completely asleep, or if you'll be in a lot of pain, or if you'll even wake up.

I hope this book has provided some useful information about what we do and what we offer. I hope it allays some common fears and provides you with a starting point for asking questions of your anesthesiologist. Writing it has reminded me of the fear that most patients have. It has reminded me how *I* felt when *I* was a surgical patient. And it has reminded me of the privilege it is to take care of you. Ask whatever questions you have. Get comfortable with me. We're going to spend some time together, after all.

Once, the thought of an anesthetic was frightening. Maybe now it can be a little less so. I hope this has been helpful. Thank you for reading.

All the best.

Brent Stewart, MD, MBA

Disclaimer of Warranty and Limit of Liability

- The author and publisher make no representations or warranties with respect to the accuracy of the contents of this work and do hereby specifically and expressly disclaim all warranties, including without limitation, warranties of title, merchantability, fitness for a particular purpose and non-infringement. No warranty may be created or extended by sales or promotional material associated with this work.

- The material contained within this work should not be attributed to any of the author's previous or present colleagues, nor to any previous or present facility at which the author held or currently holds privileges to administer anesthesia.

- Any advice, strategies, and ideas contained herein may not be suitable for particular situations. This work is sold with the understanding that the publisher is not engaging in or rendering medical advice or other professional services. If professional assistance is required, the services of a competent professional person should be sought.

- Although the author and publisher have made every effort to ensure that the information in this book was correct at press time, the author and publisher do not assume and hereby disclaim any responsibility or liability whatsoever to the fullest extent allowed by law to any party for any and all direct, indirect, incidental, special, or consequential damages, or lost profits that result, either directly or indirectly, from the use and application of any of the contents of this book. The purchaser or reader of this book alone assumes the risk for anything learned from this book.

- This book is not intended as a substitute for the medical advice of physicians and should not be used in such manner. The reader should regularly consult a physician in matters relating to his/her health and particularly with respect to any symptoms that may require diagnosis or medical attention. No guarantees of surgical or anesthetic outcomes are implied or should be inferred. Neither this text nor its author should be considered a surrogate for the reader's present surgical or anesthetic needs. Furthermore, the use of this book does not establish a doctor-patient relationship.

- The information provided in this book is designed for educational and informational purposes only and is not intended to serve as medical advice. This book is not meant to be used, nor should it be used, to diagnose or treat any medical condition. For diagnosis or treatment of any medical problem, consult your own physician. The publisher and author are not responsible for any specific health or allergy needs that may require medical supervision and are not liable for any damages or negative consequences from any treatment, action, application or preparation, to any person reading or following the information in this book.

- References are provided for informational purposes only and do not constitute or imply endorsement, sponsorship, or recommendation of any websites or other sources. Readers should be aware that the websites listed in this book may change.

- The views expressed herein are solely those of the author and do not reflect the opinions of any other person or entity.

CPSIA information can be obtained at www.ICGtesting.com
Printed in the USA
LVOW101036201012

303664LV00006B/79/P